Early Intervention Programs for Infants

Early Intervention Programs for Infants

Editors
Howard A. Moss, Robert Hess, and Carolyn Swift

Prevention in Human Services
Volume 1, Number 4

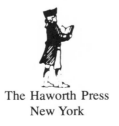

The Haworth Press
New York

The Haworth Press, Inc., 28 East 22 Street, New York, NY 10010

Library of Congress Cataloging in Publication Data
Main entry under title:

Early intervention programs for infants.

(Prevention in human services ; v. 1, no. 4)
Includes bibliographies.
Contents: Interaction coaching for high-risk infants and their parents / Tiffany Field—Mother-infant interaction and child development after rooming-in: comparison of high-risk and low-risk mothers / Susan O'Connor...[et al.]—Psychosocial change in risk groups: implications for early identification / Richard Q. Bell, David Pearl—[etc.]
1. Infants—Mental health services—Addresses, essays, lectures. 2. Infant psychiatry—Addresses, essays, lectures. 3. Child psychopathology—Prevention—Addresses, essays, lectures. I. Moss, Howard A. II. Hess, Robert, 1948- . III. Swift, Carolyn F. IV. Series.
RA790.A1C533 vol. 1, no. 4   362'.0424s   82-15608
[RJ502.5]   [362.2'0425]
ISBN 0-917724-54-2

Early Intervention Programs for Infants

Prevention in Human Services
Volume 1, Number 4

CONTENTS

Early Intervention Programs for Infants

INTRODUCTION

Prevention is a valued currency in today's health market. That it is hailed simultaneously as the health strategy of conservative government and the cherished reform of liberal health ideology testifies to its power as a concept. Prevention is an integral part of a ''paradigm shift'' taking place today in the fields of health and behavior. Such a shift changes the way scientists view the world, permitting new approaches to the resolution of problems, and the reordering of former givens. The reformulation of old questions results in an expansion of knowledge built on the former paradigm.

The capacity of the concept of prevention to encompass divergent views is rooted in the universal appeal of its goal: to reduce the incidence of human dysfunction. Its power to fuel a revolution in the health and behavioral sciences lies in the expansion of territory it claims for change. Traditionally the individual has been the target of efforts to improve the human condition. A gathering momentum targets the environment as the frontier where conquest promises the greatest return in health and happiness for increments of effort.

Prevention has an established record of progress through both individual and environmental change. Targeting the individual for change—as in innoculations and skill building—is a philosophical approach solidly in the tradition of Western political thought and psychological practice. Less frequently attempted preventive interventions have focused on changing environmental conditions—as in banning lead-based paint, draining swamps, flouridating water, and zoning residential areas against noise or chemical pollution. Having a foot in both camps—targeting both populations and environments for change—accounts for the breadth of prevention's appeal.

Prevention is consistent with a long standing tradition of developmental psychology—to use scientific information for devising guidelines to structure and facilitate an optimal developmental course for all children. Prevention is a more focused emphasis of this tradition that concentrates on that segment of the childhood population which is statistically at greater risk for behavioral dysfunction. Thus, the issues of risk and prevention are inextricably intertwined. Information concerning the course of normal development is directly relevant for intervention programs and studies of prevention significantly contribute to the theoretical understanding of early development.

Although the papers included in this volume focus on the issues of risk and prevention, the ideas and information presented have implications for generalization well beyond these issues. Models are explicated for studying the interaction of factors that contribute to behavior. Attention is given to serial and systems effects, methodological issues, research strategies, and practical problems in field research. There is a heightened consciousness of how findings obtained in the laboratory have application to real life events.

Some of the risk producing conditions dealt with in this volume include parental characteristics, socioeconomic status, infant health status, differential vulnerabilities, environmentally produced stress, and societal complacency in the responsible monitoring of critical conditions for the optimal care of infants. Attention is given not only to primary risk conditions, but to the "ripple effect" of adverse circumstances contributing to increased risk of psycho-social difficulties in other areas of the individual's life and/or social network.

The unique contribution of the set of papers gathered in this volume is their singular unanimity in transcending the traditional person-environment dichotomy. While the papers describe different approaches to preventing disorder in infants and children, most have elected to explore, in varying degrees, the reciprocal relationship between the developing child and the surrounding environment. The scientific question no longer addresses which of the two—child or environment—should be targeted for change, but instead incorporates both in a systems approach that explores the impact each has on the other in shaping outcome. The outcome of interest here is, of course, the development of children into healthy adults.

Tiffany Field's paper clearly demonstrates this focus. She has extended previous work done on specific social interaction paradigms with adults and low risk infants to high risk infants. By studying the interaction between infants and mothers she has identified key elements in the behavior of each that determine the behavior of the other. Based on this information she has projected a set of interventions effective in modulating arousal and improving the level of information processing in high risk infants. The research by O'Connor and her colleagues, utilizing mother-infant interactions at birth and subsequent intervals as the dependent variable, is a companion piece. By exploring the effects of early mother-infant contact on mothers screened to be at risk for maltreatment of their children, these two papers extend the work of Klaus and Kennell on the beneficial effects of early contact.

Bell and Pearl point out that the assignment of risk itself is not static, but fluctuates with the developmental level of the child and surrounding environment. They discuss how risk studies allow us to investigate disorders prospectively rather than retrospectively. However, they note many of the methodological, conceptual, and practical problems inherent in this type of research. Key problems are identifying false positives and negatives, the self-fulfilling prophesy of labeling, and the enormity of standard screening procedures. They recommend more frequent screening by service providers to pick up the developmental and ecological changes that determine transactional risk.

The heuristic value of focusing on the reciprocal relationship (between child and environment) is strikingly evident in the paper by Ramey and his colleagues. They provide an historical perspective on factors that have contributed to the heightened interest in prevention research. A thorough and systematic review of 18 exemplary prevention oriented programs directed at children, up to two years of age, at risk for deficits in cognitive development is presented. As a result of this review they conclude that more needs to be learned about the process and mechanisms of change and the secondary effects produced from intervention. They point to three "major new theoretical emphases or perspectives" that could enhance future infant program development: the bidirectional influence of mother-child interactions, transactional processes, and general systems theory.

Seifer and Sameroff apply structural equation model techniques to project the effects of child and background variables on child competence. They conclude that—at least in children under four—background variables contribute more to outcome than child variables.

The paper by Laskin and Pilot broadens the systems perspective to take in the wider environment outside the mother-infant pair or the home. It presents a sobering view of the bureaucratic bungling that exposed thousands of infants to defective formula. The authors' crusade brought about true systems change through their determined pursuit of rational policy at both the federal and private levels.

The final paper turns the systems approach inside out by focusing on the reciprocal effects of the prevention interventions themselves on the families and community agencies involved. In a rare, candid analysis, Rolf and his colleagues document the unexpected developments that emerge in any project designed to impact families and agencies within a community. Their project included prospective studies of children of mentally disordered parents, preventive interventions for normally behaving high risk preschoolers, and large scale surveys of the developmental competencies and behavior problems among preschoolers. In the course of their work they became cognizant of conflict between scientific, methodological, and ethical standards. From their experience they review a number of practical problems that emerged and discuss a series of risks to the staff, children, and their families that arose from participating in prevention research.

Howard Moss
Robert Hess
Carolyn Swift

INTERACTION COACHING
FOR HIGH-RISK INFANTS
AND THEIR PARENTS

Tiffany Field

ABSTRACT. This paper includes a review of literature on early interaction behaviors of infants and how they compare to adult interaction behaviors, interactions of high-risk infants and their parents, relationships of early interactions to later development, and various manipulations of early interactions. Data are then presented on interaction coaching techniques used with 60 middle income mothers of preterm infants who experienced respiratory distress syndrome. Manipulations which effectively diminished the activity levels of these extremely active mothers and enhanced their infants' visual attentiveness during interactions included mother imitation of all infant behaviors, repetition of phrases, and silencing during infants' pauses. Manipulations which were effective in increasing the amount of mother activity and the amount of infant visual attentiveness among a subsample of mothers who were very inactive were attention-getting and gameplaying manipulations. These results are discussed in the context of facilitating information processing and arousal modulation abilities of high-risk infants.

As adults we are very cognizant of our abilities to interact socially with our peers. The inability to interact effectively and the resultant social rejection, isolation and loneliness are probably dreaded more than any other life experience. Yet we know very little about the development of social interaction skills and even less about strategies to facilitate interaction skills. In this paper, some of our attempts to facilitate early interactions will be reviewed along with some of the studies by others who inspired this research.

Dr. Field is Associate Professor of Pediatrics and Psychology at the University of Miami, Miami, FL 33101.

I would like to thank the infants and mothers who participated in these studies and the research assistants who assisted with data collection. This research was aided by a social and behavioral sciences research grant form the National Foundation-March of Dimes and by grants from the Administration of Children, Youth, and Families, HEW, OHD 0090C1-764-01 and 90-C-1964(2). Requests for reprints may be mailed to the author at the Department of Pediatrics, University of Miami Medical School, PO Box 016820, Miami, FL 33101.

Similarities between Social Interaction Behaviors of Infants and Adults

During the last decade dozens of studies have been conducted on the social interactions of infants (usually with adult partners) and interactions between adults. Parallels between the descriptions of adult and infant interaction behaviors suggest that the basic interaction behaviors may be present from birth, and social experiences may contribute to their elaboration and refinement. For example, gaze alternation patterns described by Kendon (1967) and by Jaffe and Feldstein (1970) for adults are similar to those described for infants by Stern (1974). Turn-taking and signals for turn-taking described by Duncan and Fiske (1977) for adults are similar to the turn-taking behaviors of infants described by Brazelton and his colleagues (Brazelton, Koslowski, & Main, 1974). Grimacing and gesturing described for both infants and adults by Trevarthen (1975) in his lovely slide show of Henry Kissinger and an infant and affective displays described for both infants and adults by Oster and Ekman (1978) and by Field (1981b) highlight the similarities between infant and adult social interaction behaviors. Even directional changes in tonic heart rate of infants are noted to parallel those of adults during early interactions (Field, 1979b).

In addition, infants and adults appear to respond very similarly to disturbances or perturbations of interactions. Chapple (1970), for example, has described two of the most disturbing adult-adult interaction patterns, that of "interrupting" and that of "latent responding." Chapple (1970) demonstrated these disturbances in laboratory manipulations. For the demonstrations of "interrupting," the experimenter continued to make initiations to the subject without letting the subject "get a word in edgewise" which ultimately eventuated in the subject's inactivity. In the "latent responding" manipulation, the experimenter remained silent, unresponsive, or slow to respond which was increasingly stressful for the subject who continued to make initiations to the experimenter without response and ultimately became inactive.

Similar manipulations have been tried with infants and mothers. A number of researchers have manipulated early interactions in various ways such as asking the mother to remain still or stone-faced (Fogel, Diamond, Langhorst, & Demos, 1981; Trevarthen, 1974; Tronick, Als, Adamson, Wise, & Brazelton, 1978). As in the nonresponsive experimenter condition of the adult study by Chapple (1970), the infants were stressed by a nonresponsive partner as evidenced by excessive gaze aversion and fussing. The mother, like the "slow to respond" experimenter in Chapple's study, was probably equally as stressed. Similarly, some have presented a "non-stop, stimulating" mother to the infant by merely asking her to "keep her infant's attention" (Field,

1977). The mother in this situation no longer attends to her infant's gaze signals and "interrupts" the activity of the infant, eventuating in infant gaze aversion and nonresponsivity.

Interactions of High-Risk Infants and their Parents

Experiments in nature or naturalistic observations of high-risk infant/mother dyads and high-risk mother/infant dyads suggest that these types of interactions occur naturally with some frequency. For example, mothers of preterm infants have been noted to be extremely active or controlling and their infants verbally inactive and gaze averting during early interactions (Brown & Bakeman, 1979; Field, 1977, 1979b; Goldberg, Brachfeld, & DiVitto, 1980). These interactions simulate the "interrupting" experimenter situation of Chapple (1970). Conversely, lower SES mothers have been observed to be extremely inactive (or slow to respond as in the Chapple situation of latent responding) and their infants verbally inactive and gaze averting during early interactions (Bee, VanEgeren, Streissguth, Nyman, & Lockie, 1969; Field, 1980; Field, Widmayer, Stringer, & Ignatoff, 1980; Tulkin & Kagan, 1972). During these interactions there appears to be not only a relationship between the observable behaviors of the mother and infant but also parallels between unobservable but measurable physiological responses, i.e., elevated heart rate and blood pressure levels, of both mothers and infants (Field, 1979b, 1980; Field et al., 1980).

Face-to-face interactions of preterm lower SES infants (Brown & Bakeman, 1979) and preterm as well as post-term infants (Field, 1977) have been characterized by overstimulating, controlling behavior on the part of the mothers. Again, much of this overactivity probably related to their attempts to engage their fairly unresponsive infants. Pre- and post-term infants in the Field (1977) study were fussy and averted gaze for prolonged periods, and their mothers' overactive attempts to engage them in conversations were counter-productive. Interactions of these infants with their fathers as well as with sensitive experimenters revealed similar behaviors (Field, 1978).

Downs' syndrome infants engage in less eye contact, initiate fewer interaction sequences and vocalize for prolonged periods, allowing their mothers "no more than a second between breaths to respond" (Jones, 1977). In turn, their mothers are more active and "controlling." Again, the disturbed way in which each of the interactants relates to the other eludes the investigator's attempts to sort out who is to blame in this "chicken and egg" situation (Jones, 1977).

A number of investigators have reported interaction disturbances among dyads in which one member is blind. Whether the mother is blind or the infant (Als, Tronick, & Brazelton, 1980; Fraiberg, 1974), the absence of eye-to-eye contact and visual signals impairs the interaction. Fraiberg (1974) reported that interactions between blind infants and their parents could only be facilitated by teaching the parents to read the infant's hand signals.

Retrospective studies of films taken in the infancy of children later diagnosed as schizophrenic or autistic provide another source of data on disturbed interactions. Although it is often easier retrospectively to find the precursors of a condition once it has been diagnosed, many of the interaction patterns seen in the infancies of autistic and schizophrenic children are similar to the patterns already described for handicapped and developmentally at-risk infants. Analyses of infant films of twins, one of whom was later diagnosed as autistic, show lesser responsivity of both the autistic twin and his mother (Kubicek, 1980). Similarly, infant gaze avoidance and irritability behaviors, as well as over-active and controlling parent behaviors, were revealed in a retrospective analysis of home movies of infants who later were diagnosed as schizophrenic (Massie, 1980). Studies of failure-to-thrive or "atypical" infants suggest similar disturbances (Greenberg, 1971). In the case of these retrospective studies the disturbed interaction outcomes were apparent prior to the analyses of infant precursor behaviors.

Relationship of Early Interaction to Later Development

In most of the prospective studies·of high-risk infants, it is yet too soon to determine whether interaction differences predict later interaction or developmental differences. Nonetheless, there are a number of recent studies which suggest that the differences seen in high-risk infant interactions are not confined to the neonatal or early infancy periods.

Follow-up studies of preterm infants, for example, suggest that those who show interaction disturbances early in infancy experience difficulties later in infancy. In one longitudinal study, infants performing at lower levels · on sensorimotor assessments at nine months had experienced less mutual gazing at one month, fewer interchanges of smiling during gazing, and less contingent responses to distress at three months, as well as less general attentiveness and contingent responses to non-distress vocalizations at eight months (Beckwith, Cohen, Kopp, Parmelee, & Marcy, 1976). In the two year longitudinal follow-up of this group of preterm infants, the best predictor of developmental status at two years was the pattern of interaction observed during the first few months (Sigman et al., 1981). Similarly, Bakeman and

Brown (1981) report that interactions as early as three months are significantly correlated with teacher ratings of peer interactions as late as three years.

Our data suggest that the mothers who were more active and less sensitive to their infants' gaze signals at four months issued more imperatives and were over-protective or controlling during interactions at two years. The preterm infants of these mothers showed more gaze averting and fussiness at four months and manifested behavioral problems such as hyperactivity, short attention span and language production delays at two (Field, 1979b) and three years (Field, Dempsey, & Shuman, 1981). For other high-risk infants Jones (1977), reporting on Down's syndrome infants, and Kogan (1980), reporting on cerebral palsied children, suggest similar continuities.

For lower SES children (Clarke-Stewart, 1973), continuities between early interactions and later development have also been observed. Dunn (1977) has suggested that mothers' speech to the infant at 13 months is positively associated with the children's IQ scores on the Stanford-Binet at 4½ years. Further, Pawlby and Hall (1980) have reported significant correlations between the frequency of early interactions between lower SES mothers and infants and the three year language and speech development of the infants. Thus, there is some disconcerting evidence for continuity between early interaction disturbances and later developmental delays.

Rationale for Manipulating Early Interactions

Because there appear to be some continuities between early and later interaction behaviors or at least between early interaction behaviors and later language behavior, and because a number of high-risk infants show disturbances in early interactions, there may be reason to provide early interventions to facilitate early interactions. Some researchers argue that we know too little about the source of disturbance or effective manipulations to provide early intervention. This is reminiscent of the psychoanalyst's position that behavior cannot be modified until the source of the problem is well understood. Because the adult's behavior is more readily manipulated than the infant's behavior, attempts to understand the disturbed interaction have focused on the adult.

Some authors have speculated about the frequently observed hyperactivity of the mothers of unresponsive infants labelled ''at-risk'' due to perinatal complications and/or handicapping conditions. The most vague interpretation suggests that the ''frustration'' of receiving minimal responses from the infant leads to a kind of "aggressivity" on the part of the mother. Berkowitz (1974) has suggested that aggressivity often occurs in an aroused person who is presented with an aversive stimulus or a stimulus perceived to be aversive. The relative unresponsiveness of the preterm infant, his relatively less developed repertoire of coos and smiles, his frequent gaze aversion and fussiness may be perceived as aversive by the mother, as might the often noted "fragile" features of the preterm infant. In addition, the "difficult" temperaments of these infants (as evaluated by the parents; Field, Hallock, Dempsey, & Shuman, 1978) may have contributed to a parental perception of these infants as being somewhat aversive. All of these aversive factors may be generalized by the parents to even those situations when the infant is not displaying aversive behaviors such as gaze aversion and fussiness. Thus, infants viewed as aversive may simply elicit more aggressive behaviors from their parents. Another notion is that the mothers are more active to compensate for the relative inactivity of their infants, perhaps "to keep some semblance of an interaction going." A third interpretation relates to the mother wanting her child to perform like his agemates and attempting to encourage performance by more frequent modeling of behaviors. Still another explanation offered is that the mothers view their infants as fragile and delayed and, as a result, tend to be overprotective. Overprotectiveness in the extreme is construed as overcontrolling behavior. Since these infants appear to be less responsive than their normal counterparts, parents may need to work harder at generating responses such as attention, smiles, and contented vocalizations. The problem relates to finding the optimal level of stimulation, since low levels do not seem to arouse or elicit responses from these infants while high levels eventuate in gaze aversion and fussiness. Because of the seemingly higher thresholds to stimulation noted in preterm infants (Field, Dempsey, Ting, Hatch, & Clifton, 1979), Downs' syndrome infants (Cicchetti & Sroufe, 1978), and retarded infants (Kogan, 1980), the stimulation requirements may be greater for these infants than those of normal infants. But, since these infants are also more difficult to console once thresholds are exceeded (and fussing and crying ensue), the parent may be dealing with a more limited zone of optimal stimulation than are the parents of the normal infant. Although direction of effects or causality cannot be derived from these studies of early interactions, the data have evoked considerable concern since the behaviors of these dyads appear to persist beyond the period of the early interactions.

Although the continuity of early and later interaction disturbances remains uncertain, some have investigated interaction coaching techniques which might, at least, facilitate those interactions occurring during early infancy.

Interaction Coaching

Interaction coaching is a term used for attempts to modify disturbed interactions (Field, 1978). A number of manipulations have been recently tried to facilitate early interaction. They have typically been directed at the enhancement of behaviors often seen in more harmonious, synchronous interactions. The basic assumption is that the absence or infrequency of harmonious interaction behaviors in the dyad may be contributing to the disturbance. For example, if harmonious feedings typically feature the infant gazing at the mother while vigorously sucking, and the mother silently watching, reserving her words for the infant's breaks from sucking, then a disturbed feeding interaction might be characterized by a fussy, distracted, slow-to-suck, gaze-averting infant and a constantly coaxing-to-feed mother. Similarly, face-to-face interactions typically feature mothers "infantizing" or slowing down, exaggerating and repeating their behaviors, contingently responding by imitating or highlighting the infant's behaviors, taking turns or not interrupting, and respecting the infant's occasional break from the conversation, and the infant typically looking attentive and sounding content. The atypical or disturbed interaction might feature instead a gaze-averting, squirming, fussing infant and a mother who appears to be somewhat overactive, intrusive, controlling, and frustrated.

Since mothers' or adults' behaviors are more amenable to change than are the infants' behaviors, attempts to modify interactions have typically focused on altering the adults' behaviors. Manipulations, such as asking the mother to remain stone-faced or show her profile instead of her face during face-to-face interaction, dramatically demonstrate the effects of adult behavior on the infant (Stern, 1974; Tronick et al., 1978). The infant typically looks inquisitive, then makes several apparent attempts to engage her via greeting signals (vocalizations and hand gestures), alternately averts gaze, and finally turns to other activity such as hand play. Similarly, the infant can be "turned-off" to a conversation by asking the mother to pretend her husband is taking a home movie so she is trying to keep her infant looking at her (Field, 1977). Mothers invariably become more active, trying every trick in their repertoire to sustain the infant's eye contact. The infant, in turn, was given no time to respond, averted gaze, squirmed, and fussed for the duration of the interaction.

Facilitative manipulations have included asking the mother to count slowly to herself as she interacts (Tronick et al., 1978), asking her to imitate all of her infant's behaviors, repeat her words slowly, or be silent during her infant's sucking and looking away periods (Field, 1977, 1978). These manipulations vary in their effectiveness. However, each of them has resulted in longer periods of eye contact, fewer distress vocalizations, and less squirming on the part of the infant.

Other interventions include teaching the mother age-appropriate games, coaching her through an interaction via an ear piece microphone, and replaying videotapes for her viewing either with or without our running commentary (Field, 1978). These techniques, too, have been effective in facilitating interactions. Since most mothers who are experiencing difficult interactions with their infants are aware of and concerned about those difficulties, they are usually willing to try anything. Although the interaction coaching sessions seem to alter the mother's behaviors and the infant's responsivity such that they appear to have more harmonious interactions, the degree to which this experience carries over into their day-to-day interactions is unclear.

The state of the art is relatively undeveloped since we know very little about harmonious interactions, less about disturbed interactions, and even less about facilitative techniques. Nonetheless, the efficacy of the manipulations of interaction coaching we have tried suggests that adults can be shown a other ways to interact with their infants. Infants, in turn, show us that they too can interact in other ways.

Specific Manipulations of Interaction Behaviors

In this section, data will be presented on some of these manipulations of maternal behavior and their effects on infant behavior and the interactions of infants and mothers. These will include instructions to the mother to imitate their infant's behaviors, to repeat their own verbal expressions, and to remain silent when their infants looked away from them. These types of manipulations were intended to simplify and "slow down" the interactive behaviors of mothers. Other manipulations were intended to introduce variety and complexity in the mother's behaviors. Techniques used here included asking the mother to "keep her infant looking at her" (an attention-getting manipulation) and to play "infant games" for which examples were provided. Because all of these behaviors appear naturally during the spontaneous interactions of infants and mothers, we merely intended to increase the occurrence of these behaviors and observe the effects of these increases on the infant's behavior.

Before presenting the data on the various manipulations, we will describe the interaction situation and the dependent measures used. For all of these manipulations the infants observed were preterm infants who had experienced the respiratory distress syndrome as neonates. They averaged 34 weeks gestation, 1800 grams birthweight, and 31 days of intensive care during the neonatal stage. The rationale for investigating manipulation of the interactions of these particular infants was that they appeared to be less attentive and responsive during early interactions and their middle income mothers appeared to be overactive in their attempts to engage their infants, resulting in somewhat disturbed interactions (Field, 1977, 1979b).

The interactions of 60 infants were videotaped in an infant laboratory when the infants were approximately 3½ to 4½ months corrected age. Infants were placed in a semi-upright infant seat on a table face-to-face with their mothers who were seated approximately 18 inches from the infant. Two cameras, placed at approximately 6 feet at angles from the mother and infant and obscured by surrounding curtains, were used. Their separate images were mixed using a split screen generator, and a time generator superimposed a digital time record in seconds on the lower portion of the screen. Thus, the TV monitor featured the infant on one side of the screen and the mother on the other side to facilitate coding.

The general procedure was to first film a spontaneous interaction during which the mother was simply asked to "pretend she was at home playing with her infant." Following a 3-minute spontaneous interaction, the instructions for a 3-minute manipulation were given. The dyads were given no more than two manipulations per session. Multiple sessions and a large sample enabled the counterbalancing of the order of these manipulations to control for state changes across time spent in an infant seat.

Although a number of infant and mother behaviors were coded continuously using event recorders and Datamyte, only the data on the mother behavior being manipulated, e.g., imitation or repetition of phrases and infant gaze at mother, will be reported here.

Infant gaze at mother was considered an important dependent measure for the reason that it is the behavior over which the infant of this age has the most control, it is a behavior which indicates whether the infant is being attentive or inattentive, and its converse, gaze aversion, is an often-reported manifestation of disturbed interactions (Stern, 1971). In addition, gaze at mother during early interactions is that behavior which has most frequently related to later interactions, language, and social behavior.

Manipulations to Simplify and "Slow Down" the Behaviors of Mothers

Among the manipulations we hypothesized would simplify and "slow down" the behaviors of mothers were imitation, repetition of phrases, and silencing during infant gaze aversions. These were expected to have those effects because the mothers would presumably be attentive to their infants' reactions to these alterations in their behavior. Since attentiveness to signals of an interaction partner is critical for turntaking and since an infant's gaze signals provide feedback to the mother on whether she is providing appropriate levels of stimulation, the mother's enhanced attentiveness to infant behavior would presumably affect their interaction in a positive way.

Imitation

For this manipulation, mothers were asked to "imitate everything the baby does." Mothers of this age infant are noted to imitate their infant's behaviors with some frequency (Pawlby, 1977; Trevarthen, 1974). Although some of the mothers expressed that they felt "a bit silly imitating hiccups and cry behaviors," they otherwise did not feel uncomfortable with this activity.

The tapes were continuously coded for imitations by the mother which met the criterion of being behaviors of the same form in the same modality of the infant's behavior and which temporally occurred within three seconds of the behavior of the infant. The tapes were similarly coded for infant gaze at mother, defined as head aligned on the same horizontal and vertical plane as the mother's head. This behavior, rather than eye contact, was coded since interobserver reliabilities were higher for head than gaze direction. Mean number of seconds per interaction that these behaviors occurred was converted to proportion of interaction time to facilitate comparisons of data to other studies. For this manipulation and the others to follow, changes from mean percentage of baseline behaviors to the mean percentage of manipulation behavior were assessed for the mother and the infant by repeated measures analysis of variance. The criterion level of significance was set at $p < .05$ for all of these comparisons.

As can be seen in Table 1, although the incidence of imitative behavior on the part of the mother was relatively high during the spontaneous interactions, there was a significant increase in imitative behavior during that manipulation. The amount of infant gaze at mother, as predicted, increased significantly during the imitation manipulation.

Although the effectiveness of imitation as an "attention-getter" is not well understood, we have suggested that the infant looks longer at the mother during imitation because the imitative behaviors are more readily processed by the infant. The infant may require less "time-out" or pause periods or breaks in the conversation to process the mother's imitative behaviors, because they are, by definition, behaviors which are similar to behaviors

Table 1. Proportion of time mother and infant behaviors occurred during spontaneous and manipulated interactions.

Imitation Infant Behaviors	Mother Imitation	Infant Gaze
Spontaneous	.38	.42
Imitation	.84	.63
Repetition Mother Phrases	Mother Repetition	Infant Gaze
Spontaneous	.41	.41
Repetition	.76	.58
Silencing during Infant Gaze Away	Mother Silencing	Infant Gaze Away
Spontaneous	.68	.58
Silencing	.90	.30
Attention-getting Activity	Mother Activity	Infant Gaze
Spontaneous	.72	.43
Attention-getting	.95	.21
Gameplaying	Mother gameplaying	Infant Gaze
Spontaneous	.22	.45
Gameplaying	.58	.23

already in the infant's repertoire. Mother's imitations of infant hiccuping and crying were the only imitations that appeared to surprise the infants. According to the mothers, these are only infrequently imitated because the mothers are usually somewhat distressed by them and are attempting to comfort the infants when they are hiccuping or crying. Many of the imitations evolved into repetition or chains of the same behaviors with the mother's imitating the infant's behavior followed by the infant's repetition of his own behavior (or perhaps his imitation of the mother's imitation) as in a secondary circular reaction or in an infant game. While the underlying mechanism of mutual imitation is not well understood, the mother's imitation of her infant's behaviors is one of the most potent attention-getting and attention-sustaining interaction behaviors.

Repetition of Phrases

Studies by Fogel (1977) and Stern, Beebe, Jaffe, and Bennett (1977) demonstrated a relatively high frequency of the repetition of phrases by mothers of this age infant. Phrases such as ''hi ya, hi ya,'' ''you're so sweet, you're so sweet'' were noted in runs which sometimes varied slightly by words or by intonation, and which comprised approximately 64% of the mothers' phrases.

Thus, again, the mothers did not experience this instruction to ''repeat each thing you say'' as unusual or difficult, although some reported that they ''sometimes forgot to repeat themselves.'' This behavior was also noted to occur with some frequency during spontaneous interactions as can be seen in Table 1. The percentage figure here refers to the proportion of all verbal phrases (a phrase typically being two to three words followed by a pause) which were immediately repeated and closely approximated the initial phrase without considering intonation curves.

To be expected, the mother's repetition of phrases increased during the manipulation, and the mean proportion of interaction time the infants spent looking at the mother also increased. Again, the infants did not appear surprised by this manipulation and alteration of the mothers' behavior.

The same interpretation made for the effectiveness of imitation may apply here. The mothers, by providing a repetition of their phrases, may simplify the processing of information for the infant. Although the infant's processing of the content of phrases or the meaning of words is not well understood, at least the intonation quality and affective displays accompanying phrases may be more readily assimilated if they are repeated. An adult will naturally ''repeat himself'' when he is speaking in a foreign language and his listener appears not to understand, as if trying to facilitate the processing of information by the listener, although it is not clear that processing is actually facilitated in this way.

Longer looking by the infant during a manipulation which is presumed to simplify the information processing task of the infant is consistent with the notion we have advanced that infants look away or gaze avert when stimulation has exceeded the infant's capacity to modulate arousal or process information (Field, 1981a). We have interpreted the infant's gaze aversions, pauses, or breaks from the conversation as attempts to modulate arousal and process the information associated with the stimulation just provided.

Silencing During Pauses

The mother's silencing during the infant's pauses or looks away from the mother also occurs with some frequency during spontaneous interactions. Some have suggested that silence during infant gaze aversion is more likely to lead to renewed attentiveness of the infant, while others have suggested that activity of the mother is a more effective "attention-getter." The actual behavior is somewhat more complex. The infant appears more likely to return his gaze to the mother if she remains silent during his gaze aversion. However, if the mother does not emit a behavior immediately following the infant's gaze at her, the infant will revert to gaze averting or looking away behavior. This reverting to gaze aversion is similar to the gaze aversion behaviors noted during the still-face manipulation investigated by a number of interaction researchers (Fogel et al., 1980; Stoller & Field, 1981; Trevarthen, 1974; Tronick et al., 1978). The complexity of this sequence of behaviors requires more complex analyses such as the examination of event-lag probabilities. For the purposes of this paper we will report only the results of repeated measures analyses on percentages of time the behaviors were observed.

As can be seen in Table 1, the proportion of the pausing time that the mother remained silent increased during the manipulated situation. While causality cannot be determined, a parallel decrease was noted in the proportion of time the infant spent pausing. The percentage figure for the mother represents the percentage of infant pausing time that the mother remained silent, while the percentage figure noted for the infant is the percentage of interaction time that the infant spent looking away or pausing.

These manipulations of maternal activity, imitation, repetition of phrases, and silencing during pauses were accompanied by increases in the proportion of interaction time that the infants looked at their mothers. These behaviors of the mother may have been directly related to the increased amount of attentiveness by the infant.

Others have noted the attention-getting and attention-sustaining effects of imitations and mothers' frequent use of imitations during spontaneous interactions (Pawlby, 1977; Trevarthen, 1975). The reinforcing aspects of imitation are complex inasmuch as imitations are both contingent responses and simpler behaviors to process (i.e., they are already in the infant's repertoire). Thus, it is not clear whether the infant is responding to the contingent or simplicity properties of imitation or both of these.

Repetition of phrases by mothers is also a common interaction event (Fogel, 1977; Stern et al., 1977). Data reported by Stern et al. (1977) suggested that 64% of all mothers' phrases belong to "runs" of similar content, averaging 2½ repetitions per run. Repetitions were also noted to occur during the mother-infant interactions observed by Fogel (1977). Of these, he commented that maternal repetition served to sustain infant attention, "providing a structure for variations on a theme, increasing redundancy for the purpose of the infants' immature information processing capabilities and creating a stable level of expectancy for the infant."

Finally, for the attention-getting value of silencing during pauses, Field (1977) and Fogel (1981) have both noted that infants whose mothers persisted in talking during the infant's gazes away spent less time looking at their mothers. In the Fogel (1981) study, infants were more than twice as likely to begin gazing at the mother when she was not "expressive" than when she was expressive.

The infants' increased looking time may have related to a general reduction in the amount of vocalizing or talking by the mother. During each of the manipulations, the amount of talking by the mother decreased relative to baseline talking or talking during the spontaneous interactions. Alternatively, the infants' increased attentiveness may have related to the mothers' increased sensitivity or attentiveness to the infants' gaze signals. However, an assessment of this relationship would require a contingency analysis of the mothers' responses to alternation of gazing and gazing away behaviors. Without more complex contingency analyses, the relationship between changes in the behaviors measured can only be inferred. Nonetheless, the objective of these manipulations, namely to increase attentiveness of the infant, was accomplished. The instructions were simple and the mothers complied with these instructions with no apparent difficulty.

Similar interpretations were made for the effectiveness of each of these manipulations. The mothers' behaviors were simplified, the infants were faced with a simpler arousal modulation and information processing task and thus an increase in visual attentiveness to the mother. Other types of manipulations, for example, asking the mother to "get her infant's attention" or to engage in stimulating infant games such as "I'm gonna get you," have been noted to elicit increases in infant gazing-away or gaze aversion behaviors (Field, 1977; Field, 1979a). Those manipulations, that of "attention-getting" and gameplaying were included in our interaction coaching series. We expected that these might be effective for the interactions of mothers who were naturally very quiet and inactive during spontaneous interactions.

Attention-Getting Manipulation

Because this manipulation had been noted previously to result in excessive gaze aversion on the part of the infant (Field, 1977), it was always presented last. The mothers were simply asked to keep their infants looking at them. Most of the mothers immediately began to talk, to make funny sounds, make exaggerated facial expressions, to wave their hands about, and to move their faces to an en face position whenever the infants gaze averted. As can be seen in Table 1, there were dramatic increases in mother vocalization and decreases in infant gazing at mother. Several of the mothers playacted a movie-taking situation asking the infant to "look over here, look over here" and making clicking sounds as if taking photographs. Following this manipulation, many mothers said that they "tried every game" they could remember to keep their infants' attention. Several behaviors commonly noted during their spontaneous interactions such as imitation, silencing during pauses, were no longer present. An exception occurred for mothers who received the imitation manipulation prior to the attention-getting manipulation. Those mothers frequently imitated their infants' behaviors, as if having learned in the previous 3-minute situation that imitation was an effective attention-getting device. The mothers were generally amused by this situation but somewhat uncomfortable about the apparent disturbing effects of this manipulation on their infants.

This type of manipulation was clearly one of overstimulation for most of the infants. The mothers, in their attempts to sustain their infants' attention, provided excessive amounts of stimulation in auditory, tactile, kinesthetic, and facial expression modalities. In addition, they no longer appeared to attend to their infants' gaze signals. For example, they continued to talk and moved their faces into the line of their infants' visual regard when their infants turned away from them. We interpreted this as being distressful for the infant because it constituted a "stimulus overload" and because the infants were not given any pauses or breaks in the conversation to process the stimulation or modulate their apparently high arousal levels.

Gameplaying

A number of "infant" games or games which are frequently introduced to this age infant by their mothers and fathers appear to be part of the natural repertoire of at least American parents (Field, 1979a). These include "Tell me a story," "I'm gonna get you," "Peek-a-boo," "Pat-a-cake," and

"Itsy-bitsy spider" among others. These are typically noted to induce infant smiling and laughter. When these behaviors occur, parents often repeat them with subtle variations in content, form, or intensity. If they are too repetitive or intense or if the infants appear to become "too aroused" as manifested by rigorous laughter, gaze aversion often ensues. Gaze aversion in this context may indicate the infants' attempts to break from the interaction to modulate arousal.

Although this is a situation in which there may be many parameters to analyze, for example, the repetitiveness and intensity of the game and its effects on the infant as well as contingencies to analyze, the probability that mothers will alter or cease playing the game given a laughing (or highly aroused) infant, this analysis included only the proportion of interaction time that the mothers played the game they were instructed to play versus the proportion of time any games occurred during the spontaneous interaction and the amount of infant gazing at the mother.

The game, "I'm gonna get you," was used in this manipulation because it has been noted to be one of the most popular games of this age infant (Field, 1979a). This game involves a looming movement of the mother's head toward the infant's stomach. While moving her head, the mother says "I'm gonna get you, I'm gonna get you" several times and then jiggles her head on the infant's stomach. Invariably, repetitions of this game induce smiling and laughter in the infant.

As can be seen in Table 1, the incidence of playing this game was greater during the manipulation than all mother-initiated games during the spontaneous interaction. In turn, as expected, the infants engaged in less gazing at the mother, although the incidence of their affective displays (e.g., smiling and laughing) was considerably elevated during this manipulation. The increase in affective behaviors such as smiling and laughing may have increased the arousal levels of the infants. Had the mothers varied the game or its intensity or simply paused for periods of time between games, the infants may have had sufficient time to modulate their arousal. However, in compliance with the instructions to repeat the game, mothers persisted in playing the same game. Although the infants may have habituated to the particular game, "I'm gonna get you," it appeared rather that their high arousal levels derived from their being given no pauses or breaks in the repetitions of the game.

Although most of the infants showed more gaze averting behavior during the "attention-getting" and gameplaying manipulations, there were approximately 11 of 60 infants who showed increases in gazing at mother behavior during these manipulations. When we examined the spontaneous interactions of these infants and their mothers, we noted that the mothers were silent or inactive during most of the interaction time (M = 61%). During these manipulations, they became more active (M = 63% for the attention-getting manipulation and 58% for the gameplaying manipulation). Thus, although these manipulations typically served to increase the activity levels of the mothers and decrease their infants' visual attentiveness in this sample of preterm infants and their mothers, there were some dyads in which mother activity was typically low and for which the increase in mothers' activity level, apparently facilitated by these manipulations, appeared to contribute to an increase in infant attentiveness. This result highlights the need to first assess the baseline interactions of the individual dyad. While belonging to a group of middle income mothers of preterm, RDS babies, who have been noted to be extremely active during interactions (Field, 1977), these 11 mothers were clearly less active than the larger group. The earlier manipulations for simplifying and slowing down the activity of these mothers who were already extremely inactive would have clearly been inappropriate and ineffective. In this same vein, careful consideration in tailoring individual interaction coaching techniques for mothers of high-risk infants must be given to socioeconomic and cultural group differences. Dramatic differences in early interactions have been observed both within and across cultures (Field & Widmayer, 1981), even among groups who have similar native language and life-styles (Field & Pawlby, 1980).

While the manipulations used in these interaction coaching sessions were effective and were well-received by the infants' mothers, it is not clear whether any of these "games," as they were referred to by the mothers, were used during their daily interactions. Nonetheless, these data suggest that mothers and high-risk infants can be taught other ways to interact.

REFERENCES

Als, H., Tronick, E., & Brazelton, T. B. Stages of early behavioral organization: The study of a sighted infant and a blind infant in interaction with their mothers. In T. Field, S. Goldberg, D. Stern, & A. Sostek (Eds.), *High-risk infants and children: Adult and peer interactions.* New York: Academic Press, 1980.

Bakeman, R., & Brown, J. Early interaction: Consequences for social and mental development at three years. *Child Development*, 1980, *51*, 437–447.

Bee, H. L., VanEgeren, L. F., Streissguth, A. P., Nyman, B. A., & Lockie, M. S. Social class differences in maternal teaching styles and speech patterns. *Developmenal Psychology*, 1969, *1*, 726–734.

Beckwith, L., Cohen, S. E., Kopp, C. Y., Parmelee, A. H., & Marcy, T. G. Caregiver-infant interaction and early cognitive development in preterm infants. *Child Development*, 1976, *47*, 579–587.

Berkowitz, L. Some determinants of impulsive aggression: Role of mediated associations with reinforcements for aggression. *Psychological Review*, 1974. *81*. 165–176.

Brazelton, T. B., Koslowski, B., & Main, M. The origins of reciprocity: The early mother-infant interaction. In M. Lewis & L. Rosenblum (Eds.), *The effect of the infant on its caregiver*. New York: Wiley, 1974.

Brown, J. M., & Bakeman, R. Relationships of human mothers with their infants during the first year of life: Effect of prematurity. In R. W. Bell & W. P. Smotherman (Eds.), *Maternal influences and early behavior*. New York: Spectrum, 1979.

Chapple, E. D. Experimental production of transients in human interaction. *Nature*, 1970, *288*, November 14.

Cicchetti, D., & Stroufe, L. A. An organizational view of affect: Illustration from the study of Downs' syndrome infants. In M. Lewis & L. A. Rosenblum, (Eds.), *The development of affect*, Vol. 1. New York: Plenum, 1978.

Clark-Stewart, K. A. Interactions between mothers and their young children: Characteristics and consequences. *Monographs of SRCD*, 1973, *38*, (6–7, Serial No. 153).

Duncan, S., & Fiske, D. W. *Face-to-face interaction: Research, methods and theory*. Hillsdale, N.J.: Lawrence Erlbaum Associates, 1977.

Dunn, J. B. Patterns of early interaction: Continuities and consequences. In H. R. Schaffer (Ed.), *Studies in mother-infant interaction*. New York: Academic Press, 1977.

Field, T. Effects of early separation, interactive deficits and experimental manipulations on infant-mother face-to-face interaction. *Child Development*, 1977, *48*, 763–771.

Field, T. The three Rs of infant-adult interactions: Rhythms, repertoires and responsivity. *Journal of Pediatrics Psychology*, 1978, *3*, 131–136.

Field, T. Games parents play with normal and high-risk infants. *Child Psychiatry and Human Development*, 1979, *10*, 41–48. (a)

Field, T. Interaction patterns of high-risk and normal infants. In T. Field, A. Sostek, S. Goldberg & H. H. Shuman (Eds.), *Infants born at risk*. New York: Spectrum, 1979. (b)

Field, T. Interactions of preterm and term infants with their lower and middle class teenage and adult mothers. In T. Field, S. Goldberg, D. Stern, & A. Sostek (Eds.), *High-risk infants and children: Adult and peer interactions*. New York: Academic Press, 1980.

Field. T. Infant gaze aversion and heart rate during face-to-face interactions. *Infant behavior and development*, 1981. (a)

Field, T. Social perception. In T. Field, A. Huston, H. Quay, L. Troll, & G. Finley (Eds.), *Review of human development*. New York: Wiley Interscience, 1981. (b)

Field, T. M., Dempsey, J. R., & Shuman, H. H. Developmental follow-up of pre- and post-term infants. In S. L. Friedman & M. Sigman (Eds.), *Preterm birth and psychological development*. New York: Academic Press, 1981.

Field, T., Dempsey, J., Ting, G., Hatch, J., & Clifton, R. Cardiac and behavioral responses to repeated tactile and auditory stimulation by preterm and fullterm infants during the neonatal period. *Developmental Psychology*, 1979, *15*, 406–416.

Field, T., Hallock, N., Dempsey, J., & Shuman, H. Mothers' assessments of term infants and preterm infants with respiratory distress syndrome: Reliability and predictive validity. *Child Psychiatry & Human Development*, 1978, *9*, 75–85.

Field, T., & Pawlby, S. Early face-to-face interactions of British and American working and middle class mother-infant dyads. *Child Development* , 1980, *51*, 250–253

Field, T., Sostek, A., Vietze, P., & Leiderman, P. H. *Culture and early interactions*. Hillsdale, N. J.: Lawrence Erlbaum Associates, 1980.

Field, T., & Widmayer, S. Mother-infant interactions among lower SES Black, Cuban, Puerto Rican, and South American immigrants. In T. Field, A. Sostek, P. Vietze, & A. H. Leiderman (Eds.), *Culture and early interactions*. Hillsdale, N.J.: Lawrence Erlbaum, 1981.

Field, T., Widmayer, S., Stringer, S., & Ignatoff, E. Teenage, lower class black mothers and their preterm infants: An intervention and developmental follow-up. *Child Development*, 1980, *51*, 426–436.

Fogel, A., Diamond, G. R., Langhorst, B. H., & Demos, V. Affective and cognitive aspects of the two-month-old's participation in face-to-face interaction with its mother. In E. Tronick (Ed.), *Joint regulation of behavior*. Cambridge, England: Cambridge University Press, 1981.

Fogel, A. The role of repetition in the mother-infant face-to-face interaction. In H .R. Schaffer (Ed.), *Studies in mother-infant interaction*. London: Academic Press, 1977.

Fogel, A. *Early adult-infant interaction: Expectable sequences of behavior*. Unpublished manuscript. Purdue University, 1981.

Fraiberg, S. Blind infants and their mothers: An examination of the sign system. In M. Lewis & L. A. Rosenblum (Eds.), *The effect of the infant on its caregiver*. New York: Wiley & Sons, 1974.

Goldberg, S., Brachfeld, S., & DiVitto, B. Feeding, fussing, and playing: Parent-infant interaction in the first year as a function of prematurity and prenatal problems. In T. Field, S. Goldberg, D. Stern, & A. Sostek (Eds.), *High risk infants and children: Adult and peer interactions*. New York: Academic Press, 1980.

Greenberg, N. H. A comparison of infant-mother interactional behavior in infants with atypical behavior and normal infants. In J. Hellmuth (Ed.), *Exceptional infant*, Vol. 2. New York: Brunner/Mazel, 1971.

Jaffe, J., & Feldstein, S. *Rhythms of dialogue*. New York: Academic Press, 1970.

Jones, O. H. M. Mother-child communication with pre-linguistic Downs' Syndrome and normal infants. In H. R. Schaffer (Ed.), *Studies in mother-infant interaction*. London: Academic Press, 1977.

Kendon, A. Some functions of gaze-direction in social interaction. *Acta Psychologica*, 1967, *26*, 22–63.

Kogan, K. L. Interaction systems between preschool aged handicapped or developmentally delayed children and their parents. In T. Field, S. Goldberg, D. Stern, & A. Sostek (Eds.), *High-risk infants and children: Adult and peer interactions*. New York: Academic Press, 1980.

Kubicek, L. Mother interactions of twins: An autistic and non-autistic twin. In T. Field, S. Goldberg, D. Stern, & A. Sostek. *High risk infants and children: Adult and peer interactions*. New York: Academic Press, 1980.

Massie, H. N. Pathologie interactions in infancy. In T. Field, S. Goldberg, D. Stern, & A. Sostek (Eds.), *High-risk infants and children: Adult and peer interactions*. New York: Academic Press, 1980.

Oster, H., & Ekman, P. Facial behavior in child development. In *Minnesota symposium on child psychology*, Vol. 11. Minneapolis: University of Minnesota Press, 1978.

Pawlby, S. Imitative interaction. In H. R. Schaffer (Ed.), *Studies in mother-infant interaction*. London: Academic Press, 1977.

Pawlby, S., & Hall, F. Early interactions and later language development of children whose mothers come from disrupted families or origin. In T. Field, S. Goldberg, D. Stern, & A.M. Sostek (Eds.), *High-risk infants and children: Adult and peer interactions*. New York: Academic Press, 1980.

Sigman, M., Cohen, S. E., & Forsythe, A. B. The relations of early infant measures to later development. In S. L. Friedman & M. Sigman (Eds.), *Preterm birth and psychological development*. New York: Academic Press, 1971.

Stern, D. N. A micro-analysis of mother-infant interaction: Behavior regulating social contact between a mother and her 3½-month-old twins. *Journal of American Academy of Child Psychiatry*, 1971, *10*, 501–517.

Stern, D. N. Mother and infant at play. In M. Lewis & L. Rosenblum (Eds.), *The effect of the infant on its caregiver*. New York: Wiley & Sons, 1974.

Stern, D., Beebe, B., Jaffe, J., & Bennett, S. L. (Eds.). The infant's stimulus world during social interaction: A study of caregiver behaviors with particular reference to repetition and timing. In H. R. Schaffer (Ed.), *Studies in mother-infant interaction*. New York: Academic Press, 1977.

Stoller, S., & Field, T. *Alteration of mother and infant behaviors and heart rate during a still-face perturbation of face-to-face interaction.* Unpublished manuscript, University of Miami, 1981.

Trevarthen, C. Conversations with a 2-month-old. *New Scientist,* 1974, *22,* 230–235.

Trevarthen, C. B. *The nature of an infant's ecology.* Paper presented at the International Society for the Study of Behavioral Development, Guildford, England, 1975.

Tronick, E., Als, H., Adamson, L., Wise, S., & Brazelton, T. B. The infant's response to entrapment between contradictory messages in face-to-face interaction. *Journal of Child Psychiatry,* 1978, *17,* 1–13.

Tulkin, S., & Kagan, J. Mother-child interaction in the first few years of life. *Child Development,* 1972, *43,* 31–41.

MOTHER-INFANT INTERACTION AND CHILD DEVELOPMENT AFTER ROOMING-IN: COMPARISON OF HIGH-RISK AND LOW-RISK MOTHERS

Susan O'Connor
Peter Vietze
Kathryn Sherrod
Howard M. Sandler
Sue Gerrity
W.A. Altemeier

ABSTRACT. One hundred and seventy-two low-income women were interviewed prenatally to determine risk for later mistreatment of their children. High-risk and low-risk women were then randomly assigned at delivery to either limited or extended postpartum contact with their newborns over the first two days after birth. Mother-infant interaction observations were performed at 48 hours and at one, three, six, twelve and eighteen months postpartum. Infants were tested at nine months with the Bayley Scales of Infant Development. Results indicated that outcome following extended mother-infant postpartum contact varies with maternal risk status and measures employed for evaluation. Low-risk extended-contact mother-infant pairs differed from low-risk controls in observed interaction while high-risk extended-contact and controls did not differ from each other in interaction. High-risk extended-contact infants were more advanced in motor development than control infants at nine months, however, while low-risk extended contact and control infants did not differ in development.

Dr. O'Connor is Assistant Professor of Pediatrics at Vanderbilt University. Dr. Vietze is Head, Mental Retardation Research Center, National Institute of Child Health and Human Development, Bethesda, MD. Dr. Sherrod is Assistant Professor of Psychology and Dr. Sandler is Associate Professor of Psychology at Peabody College, Vanderbilt University. Dr. Gerrity is a Research Associate in Pediatrics and Dr. Altemeier is Professor of Pediatrics at Vanderbilt University.

This research was supported by the William T. Grant Foundation; the National Center on Child Abuse and Neglect/Children's Bureau Administration on Children, Youth and Families grants No. 90-C-419 and 90-CA-2138; and the National Institute of Mental Health grant No. 2R01 MH 31195. Reprints may be obtained from Susan O'Connor, Department of Pediatrics, Vanderbilt University Medical Center, Nashville, TN 37232.

Hospital practice permitting postpartum rooming-in has been shown to facilitate the subsequent mother-infant relationship. Positive outcome has been documented in three randomized prospective longitudinal studies. The first of these divided 28 low-income mothers equally between control and experimental groups (Klaus, Jerauld, Kreger, McAlpine, Steffa, & Kennel, 1972; Kennel, Jerauld, Wolfe, Chesler, Kreger, McAlpine, Steffa, & Klaus, 1974; Ringler, Kennell, Jarvella, Navojosky, & Klaus, 1975). Experimental mothers received one hour of contact with their newborns during the first three postpartum hours and rooming-in five hours daily over the first three days after delivery. Control mothers were separated from their infants during the first postpartum hours and then were with them only every four hours for brief feedings. Data from observations and interviews at one and 12 months postpartum suggested that the extra contact mothers were more involved with and attached to their children. In addition, at 12 months extra contact children were more advanced in mental development on standardized tests than controls; and at two years extra contact mothers spoke to their children in a more stimulating fashion, using more adjectives and questions and fewer commands than control mothers.

The second study (Siegel, Bauman, Schaefer, Saunders, & Ingram, 1980) used the same experimental and control contact schedule and low-income women equally divided between groups. Extra postpartum mother-infant contact significantly added to the amount of variance accounted for in predicting maternal acceptance and consoling of the infant at four months and infant's positive/negative behavior at 12 months. Although significant, the amount of variance explained for these factors by extra postpartum contact was small (2–3%) and much less than that accounted for by maternal background factors such as age and education (10–22%). Both of these studies included a component of early mother-infant contact during the first three postpartum hours as well as extended contact.

The third study (O'Connor, Vietze, Sherrod, Sandler, & Altemeier, 1980) examined extended postpartum contact over the two day hospital stay, but did not include contact in the initial postpartum hours. Participants were 301 low-income women divided into rooming-in and control groups. Follow-up revealed that the rooming-in group had significantly fewer problems with inadequate parenting. Seven percent of the control children versus 1.5% of the rooming-in children suffered nonorganic failure-to-thrive, abuse, hospitalization due to inadequate parental care, neglect, or abandonment. The second phase of this investigation (O'Connor, Vietze, Altemeier, Sandler, Sherrod, Falsey, Gerrity, & Hopkins, Notes 1–3) explored the mechanisms by which rooming-in might influence parenting. Mother-infant interaction to 18 months after rooming-in versus limited postpartum mother-infant contact was compared. Results suggested that rooming-in facilitates early mutual regulation of mother and infant behaviors at 48 hours and one month postpartum, leading to increased variety and responsivity of interaction at six, 12, and 18 months. This pattern of mutual exchange could influence quality of parenting through positive reinforcement.

Both groups of mothers in this last study included 16% who had been classified prenatally as high-risk and 84% classified low-risk for subsequent child maltreatment using an experimental predictive interview (Altemeier, Vietze, Sherrod, Sandler, Falsey, & O'Connor, 1979; Altemeier, Vietze, Sherrod, Sandler, Tucker, & O'Connor, 1980). This interview gathers information about a mother's background currently and during her own childhood and has been shown to identify a high-risk group of pregnant women in which child abuse and neglect does occur much more frequently. For several reasons it is of interest to determine whether rooming-in affects mothers of varying backgrounds differently. First, it is of practical value to know which mothers will benefit most from extended postpartum contact with their newborns. Second, knowledge of variable effects of rooming-in upon mothers differing in past experiences may be useful in interpreting results of studies which are not comparable in sample characteristics and outcome measures. Also, this information may help to clarify the mechanisms by which rooming-in affects long term changes in the mother-infant relationship. For example, in the third study described above, results suggested that child maltreatment may be reduced by the rooming-in experience. Since women predicted to be high risk for child maltreatment were equally represented in the rooming-in and control groups, it would appear that high-risk mothers are most influenced by rooming-in. Results also indicated that rooming-in affects parenting through an intermediary influence upon the mother-infant interaction, but it is unclear whether this is equally the case for both low and high-risk mothers. The analyses reported here examined these issues by comparing consequences of rooming-in within low-risk and high-risk groups from 48 hours to 18 months postpartum.

Method

Participants

Participants were 172 mother-infant pairs divided into four groups according to risk and rooming-in conditions. There were 34 low-risk rooming-in, 36 high-risk rooming-in, 51 low-risk control, and 51 high-risk control mother-infant pairs. Participants were a subsample of a larger prospective study of antecedents of child maltreatment (Altemeier et al., 1979, 1980). For the larger study, 1489 consecutive low-income women attending the prenatal clinic at Nashville General Hospital from September, 1975, to December, 1976, were asked to participate; 1400 gave informed consent and were interviewed during the first prenatal visit to determine risk for later child abuse or neglect (see below for details of risk prediction). All of the high risk women (N=273) and a random sample of the remaining low risk women (N=225) were then selected for further study. Of these 498 selected participants, 270 actually delivered viable infants at the study hospital and met the health criteria necessary for participation in this study, and 172 of these 270 also were available at 48 hours postpartum for data collection. These 172 mother-infant pairs constitute the subjects reported here. The remaining 98 from the 270 eligible subjects were equally distributed between the four study groups and are excluded from this report because they either were discharged prior to 48 hours postpartum or had missing data sets at 48 hours due to research equipment malfunction. Participants with complete data sets at 48 hours were retained at subsequent data collection points whenever possible, although most missed at least one scheduled mother-infant interaction observation between one and 18 months postpartum.

Procedure

The criteria for actual participation in this study and the details of the rooming-in arrangement have been previously published (O'Connor et al., 1980). Briefly, to be participants the women had to remain healthy during pregnancy and have single, fullterm, well newborns delivered vaginally. Women were randomly assigned at the time of admission to rooming-in or control postpartum groups. Control mothers received a glimpse of the infant while on the delivery table and then were separated from the baby for a minimum of 12 hours; thereafter control mothers and infants were together only during feedings. The rooming-in group followed the same routine until the infant was at least seven hours old and then the newborn was placed in the mother's room for up to eight hours each day until discharge. During the first 48 hours postpartum, rooming-in mothers averaged 9.3 more hours with their infants than control mothers.

While obtaining informed consent in the prenatal clinic, study mothers were told that the investigation concerned factors which affect the mother-child relationship, but rooming-in was not mentioned. All data collectors were also unaware that rooming-in was being studied. After the hospital data collection period, research assistants were naive to subject assignment to rooming-in or control groups; throughout the investigation they were uninformed about prenatally determined subject risk status for maltreatment.

Measures

Risk assignment. During the prenatal period, study mothers were administered the Maternal History Interview (MHI) as part of the larger child abuse investigation. The MHI is an experimental instrument designed for use during pregnancy to predict women at high risk of later mistreating their children. A prior study indicated that the instrument can predict child abuse, neglect, and nonorganic failure-to-thrive to a statistically significant degree (Altemeier et al., 1979, 1980). The MHI contains questions divided into eight major categories based upon factors reported to be associated with child maltreatment: mother's feelings about her current pregnancy, support systems available, nurturance during her own childhood, current stress from drugs or health problems in the family, personality, parenting skills, expectations of child development, and the Life Stress Inventory (Holmes & Rahe, 1967). The MHI was given by trained interviewers who maintained agreement reliability of .90 or greater throughout the study period. Subjects were not informed of their risk assignment. MHI risk scores in this study were used only to examine the effects of subject attrition upon results and to identify the four experimental groups: low-risk rooming-in or control and high-risk rooming-in or control.

The Maternal Attitude Scale (Cohler, Weiss, & Grunebaum, 1970) was also administered to study women prenatally. This instrument assesses childrearing attitudes on an adaptive-maladaptive scale. Scores from this measure were used to assure that randomization equally distributed mothers with maladaptive attitudes between rooming-in and control groups.

Mother-infant interaction. Observation of mother-infant interaction was done at two days in the hospital and at one, three, six, 12, and 18 months postpartum in the homes. The hospital observations were done as close as possible to 48 hours after delivery, except when 48 hours postpartum fell between 10 p.m. and 8 a.m. In such instances, observations were done the following morning prior to discharge from the hospital. The home observations were scheduled in advance with the mothers by asking them to choose a time when their infants ordinarily were awake, contented and soon to be fed. Observations lasted 60 minutes and included a feeding. The observational system (Anderson, Vietze, Faulstich, & Ashe, 1978) utilized an Electro General Datamyte and trained observers who entered predetermined codes for the context in which interaction occurred (maternal caretaking setting, proximity to the child and infant state of arousal) and for actual maternal-infant behaviors which made up the content of their interaction. Codes for the three contextual factors were: *maternal caretaking setting* - cradling infant, feeding infant, nonfeeding caretaking, and no caretaking; *proximity to the child* - out of room, in room but distant, within arm's reach of infant, and holding; and *infant state of arousal* - sleeping, drowsy, alert, fussing, and crying. Codes within each of these three contextual factors were mutually exclusive.

Codes for mother and infant behaviors each consisted of nine mutually exclusive and exhaustive combinations of four basic behaviors and one code for no interaction. The maternal behaviors were visual attention to infant, vocalization to infant, smile at infant, and tactile play with infant; those for the infant were visual attention to mother, vocalization, cry, and smile. As each code was entered, the time in seconds from the beginning of the observation was automatically recorded. After an observation ended, the record was entered on a PDP 11/40 computer, edited, and made available for data reduction and retrieval. Comparisons between groups were made for proportion of each observation occupied by each component of the three contextual factors, by the four basic maternal and infant behaviors, and by no maternal or infant interactive behaviors expressed. This resulted in 23 comparisons of rooming-in and control within each of the two risk groups at each observation point. Interobserver reliability estimates are published (Vietze, Falsey, O'Connor, Sander, Sherrod, & Altemeier, 1980) and averaged .71.

In addition to information about the duration of behaviors from mother-infant observations, interaction data were analyzed for the probability of transition between dyadic states using a technique which has been proposed to assess the flow of mother-infant interaction (Lewis & Lee-Painter, 1974). To do this, the presence of any of the four basic behaviors from the observational records was scored as a response for the mother or infant. This converted the interaction record to a sequence of four possible dyadic states: (a) the coacting state when both are simultaneously responding; (b) mother alone; (c) infant alone; and (d) neither partner acting, the quiescent state. For example, in the *dyadic state, mother only*, the mother displayed one or a combination of looking at, talking to, smiling at, or touching her infant while the child was not looking or smiling at the mother, vocalizing, or crying. The converse of this was the *dyadic state, infant only*. In the *dyadic state, both responding* (or coacting), mother and infant were concurrently displaying one or more of the four basic interactive behaviors. In the *dyadic state, none responding*, neither partner was exhibiting interactive behavior toward the other.

A transition matrix with five second intervals was then derived using these four dyadic states, and the conditional probability of change between states was obtained from this matrix. This form of data analysis, sequential analysis through construction of a matrix of transitional probabilities (Lewis & Lee-Painter, 1974; Bakeman & Brown, 1977), computes the likelihood that maternal and infant behavior observed at time zero will be occurring at a specified time interval later, in this case five seconds. For example, if during an observational session the dyadic state, mother alone, occurs 100 times and if 25 of these times are followed five seconds later by the coacting state, then the transition probability for mother to both responding would be .25. Once the transition probability matrix was constructed for each dyad, the transitions were treated as scores and analyzed. Probability scores for the rooming-in and control groups were compared statistically to determine if they differentiated the groups.

In this report, 12 transition probabilities are used to describe responsivity of dyadic interaction of subjects. Four of these reflect maternal responsivity to the infant: contingent maternal response given (infant to both), response stops contingently (both to infant), and lack of responsiveness (infant to infant, infant to none). Four describe infant responsivity to mother: contingent infant response given (mother to both), response stops contingently (both to mother), and lack of responsiveness (mother to mother, mother to none). The four other scores describe mutuality of mother-infant responsivity: coacting continues (both to both), coacting stops (both to none), and no coacting (mother to infant, infant to mother). These last three response transitions (both to none, mother to infant, infant to mother) are very abrupt and rarely seen in normal mother-infant interaction (Bakeman & Brown, 1977; O'Connor, Altemeier, Gerrity, Sandler, & Sherrod, 1981). The latter two by definition indicate temporal separation of maternal and infant behavior since both partners are acting sequentially but in isolation.

When the infants were nine months old, they were tested by a single trained examiner using the Bayley Scales of Infant Development. Statistical analyses were done using ANOVAs. Because the variances contained in Tables 2–3 were often heterogeneous, significance levels determined by ANOVAs were confirmed by Welch's t' test (Myers, 1972; Welch, 1937) when variances were not homogeneous.

Results

As indicated in Table 1, rooming-in and control subjects within each of the two groups did not differ in maternal age, education, race, marital status, gravidity, prenatal childrearing attitudes, MHI total score or subscale scores,

Table 1

Characteristics of Subjects

	Low-Risk		High-Risk	
	Rooming-in	Control	Rooming-in	Control
Age [a] (years)	20.2 ± 4.6	21.6 ± 5.8	21.1 ± 4.4	20.8 ± 4.2
Education (years)	10.2 ± 1.8	10.4 ± 1.6	9.9 ± 2.1	10 ± 2
% Black	25%	28%	29%	31%
Marital status [b]	1.8 ± 0.6	2 ± 0.8	1.9 ± 0.9	1.9 ± 0.8
# Pregnancies	0.6 ± 2.0	0.5 ± 1.9	2.4 ± 1.7	2.52 ± 1.3
Childrearing attitudes	135 ± 23	136 ± 21	132 ± 21	129 ± 27
MHI: Total score [c]	3.0 ± 0.7	3.2 ± 0.7	4.0 ± 0.5	4.1 ± 0.7
MHI: Pregnancy attitude	1.98 ± 5.6	1.34 ± 5.2	-3.23 ± 7.1	-2.88 ± 6.5
MHI: Support systems	2.65 ± 4.2	2.42 ± 4.3	-1.66 ± 5.5	-1.41 ± 6.1
MHI: Nurturance	-0.27 ± 7.6	-0.79 ± 6.8	-12.75 ± 13	-10.49 ± 11.7
MHI: Stress	-0.73 ± 2.2	-1.04 ± 2.4	-3.52 ± 2.8	-3.44 ± 2.8
MHI: Personality	0.54 ± 5.0	0.76 ± 4.2	-4.54 ± 5.8	-4.51 ± 5.0
MHI: Parenting skills	0.40 ± 2.8	0.68 ± 2.3	-2.36 ± 4.1	-2.62 ± 4.3
Infant birthweight (grams)	2334	2324	3340	3315

[a]
Numbers are means unless otherwise indicated.

[b]
1 = married, 2 = single, 3 = divorced, 4 = separated

[c]
Higher MHI total scores = higher risk. For the MHI subscales, however, lower score = higher risk.

and infant birthweight. Half of the infants in each group were males. High-risk subjects, regardless of rooming-in or control status, differed from low-risk subjects by having been more often pregnant and by delivering larger infants. The extreme MHI scores in the high risk group were anticipated by definition.

Attrition

Despite extensive efforts to avoid subject attrition, (O'Connor et al., Note 1), only half of the initial sample remained with the study to 18 months postpartum. To evaluate the possible effects of attrition upon interpretation of the results, a series of 2 (rooming-in vs. control) × 2 (lost vs. retained) × 2 (high-risk vs. low-risk) ANOVAs were computed, using presence in the eighteen month data set as the criterion for retained subjects. Twenty-four independent variables were examined: mother's age, education, race, number of children and pregnancies, parity, marital status, pregnancy or delivery complications, intention to breastfeed, and MHI subscale scores; infant's birthweight, sex, gestational age, one minute Apgar, and nursery complications. For variables such as race and marital status, "dummy" numerical codes were assigned so that ANOVAs could be used for statistical comparisons. No differences which might have artifactually influenced results were found. Subjects who dropped out of the study, regardless of risk status or rooming-in/control assignment, had fewer years of education [9.9 vs. 10.5, $F (1,219) = 5.691, p < .05$] and fewer nursery complications [$F (1,262) = 5.643, p < .05$] than those who remained. (Nursery complications were minor since all study subjects met the criteria of health necessary for inclusion in the investigation.) More black mothers remained with the study than dropped out [$F (1,262) = 9.215, p < .01$]. Only two significant interactions between risk, treatment assignment, and attrition were found in this series of analyses, and one-way ANOVAs were computed to determine wherer the interaction occurred. The first interaction concerned race and risk status of the subjects. Of all women staying with the study, there were more low-risk blacks than high-risk blacks [$F (1,85) = 2.08, p = .05$]; within the low-risk group, black subjects more often stayed in the study than dropped out [$F (1,126) = 2.196, p < .01$]. The other interaction concerned treatment group assignment and attrition. Compared to rooming-in mothers lost to follow-up, rooming-in mothers remaining with the study had more negative feelings about their pregnancy as measured prenatally by MHI scores, [$F (1,107) = 3.76, p < .01$]. Rooming-in and control mothers remaining with the study did not differ on this MHI subscale. While attrition may have influenced outcome other than through these independent variables, there is little evidence from the measures which were gathered to indicate artifacts in results.

Tables 2 and 3 indicate results for maternal mode of caretaking, proximity to the infant, infant state, and specific maternal and infant interactive behaviors expressed in percentage of observed time. All comparisons are between rooming-in and control groups with risk held constant.

When findings within a risk group are few, they appear in the text and not in the Tables. Statistics for comparisons differing at the .05 level of confidence appear in Tables 2 and 3 while those for trends appear in the text.

Forty-eight Hours Postpartum

Low-risk. In the low-risk group there was only one difference between rooming-in and control; rooming-in infants spent more time sleeping [36% vs. 24%, $F (1,83) = 4.83, p < .05$].

High-risk. High-risk rooming-in infants also tended to sleep more [31% vs. 21%, $F (1,85) = 3.39, p < .10$]. High-risk rooming-in mothers devoted more time to non-feeding infant caretaking (Table 2) and spent more time only within arm's reach of their infants, while high-risk control mothers held their infants more. High-risk infants showed no differences in basic interactive behaviors between the two groups. High-risk groups, however, differed on almost all maternal behaviors. High-risk control mothers looked at their infants more (Table 2), touched them more, and tended to smile at their infants more [8% vs. 5%, $F (1,85) = 2.93, p < .10$]. High-risk rooming-in mothers tended to spend more time not interacting with their newborns [16% vs. 11%, $F (1,85) = 3.31, p < .10$].

One to Eighteen Months Postpartum

Low-risk. Results will be presented in the text in chronological order, while, for brevity, data are presented in Table 3 by categories with infant age indicated in parentheses on the right. At one month, rooming-in children were more drowsy while control infants cried more. Control mothers tended to spend more time entirely out of the room containing the infant [2% vs. 3%, $t'(54) = 1.937, p < .10$] and when in the same room spent more

Table 2

Mother-Infant Interaction 48 Hours After Delivery: High-Risk Sample

	Rooming-in (N=36)	Control (N=51)	F/t' (df)
Mother:			
Performs nonfeeding caretaking	5.65(7.85)[a]	1.18(4.92)**	$F(1,85) = 10.66$
Is only in arm's reach of infant	19.43(22.3)	8.73(16.9)*	$F(1,85) = 6.47$
Holds infant	80.4(22.4)	91.16(17.2)*	$F(1,85) = 6.44$
Looks at infant	81.15(19.86)	88.68(10.57)*	$t'(36) = 2.077$
Touch plays with infant	1.30(2.13)	3.14(6.05)*	$t'(66) = 2.003$

[a] Numbers are percentages of observed time followed by standard deviations in parentheses.

*$p < .05$ **$p < .01$

time physically distant from their infants. At three months, control infants slept more and tended to fuss more [16% vs. 9%, $t'(51) = 1.735, p < .10$]. Control mothers spent more time distant from their infants and tended to look at their infants less [71% vs. 82%, $t'(11) = 1.82, p < .10$]. At six months, control infants were more drowsy and tended to cry more [3% vs. 0.5%, $t'(27) = 1.711, p < .10$], while rooming-in children spent more time alert. Control mothers tended to be more physically distant from their infants, i.e., entirely out of the room [8% vs. 1%, $t'(27) = 1.841, p < .10$], looked at their infants less, and spent more time not interacting with their children. Rooming-in children tended to look at their mothers more [28% vs. 21%, $F(1,39) = 3.5, p < .10$]. At 12 months, control mothers tended to spend more time in activities unrelated to their infants' physical care [54% vs. 38%, $F(1,34) = 3.48, p < .10$]. Rooming-in mothers smiled at their children more, while control mothers tended to spend more time not interacting with their children [26% vs. 13%, $F(1,34) = 3.66, p < .10$]. Rooming-in children tended to vocalize more [32% vs. 26%, $F(1,34) = 2.94, p < .10$] and spent less time not interacting with their mothers. At 18 months, rooming-in mothers smiled at their children more.

High-risk. At one month, control mothers tended to be more physically distant from their children, out of the room entirely [3% vs. 1%, $t'(83) = 1.706, p < .10$] or in the room but not within arm's reach [6% vs. 2%, $t'(75) = 1.895, p < .10$]. At three months, rooming-in mothers tended to feed their infants more [40% vs. 29%, $t'(33) = 1.854, p < .10$] but control mothers tended to smile at their children more [10% vs. 5%, $t'(70) = 1.73, p < .10$]. No differences were found at six months. At 12 and 18 months, control mothers again were more distant from their children, not within arm's reach [25% vs. 5% at 12 months, $t'(44) = 4.876, p < .001$; 21% vs. 9% at 18 months, $F(1,44) = 4.88, p < .05$] while rooming-in mothers held their children more at 18 months [39% vs. 16%, $F(1,44) = 8.63, p < .01$]. At 12 months, control children tended to vocalize more [27% vs. 20%, $F(1,53) = 3.24, p < .10$], while at 18 months rooming-in children tended to look at their mothers more [27% vs. 21%, $F(1,44) = 3.12, p < .10$].

Responsivity During Mother-Infant Interaction

Low-risk. Probabilities for response transitions for low-risk rooming-in and control groups are compared in Table 4. Results are presented in the text in chronological order but appear in the Table by category. At one month, control mothers were more likely not to respond to their infants (in-

Table 3

Mother-Infant Interaction from One to Eighteen Months Postpartum: Low-Risk Sample[a]

Factor	Rooming-in	Control	F/t' (df)
Infant state:			
Sleeping	1.57[b] (3.14)	5.49* (9.2)	t'(46) = 2.276 (3 months[c])
Drowsy	35.39 (27)	23.78* (23.5)	F (1,76) = 3.99 (1 month)
	0.35 (1.1)	6.83* (14.94)	t'(25) = 2.201 (6 months)
Alert	88.76 (16.7)	71.67* (31.3)	t'(39) = 2.278 (6 months)
Crying	0.32 (0.98)	2.76* (7.75)	t'(51) = 2.175 (1 month)
Maternal proximity to infant:			
In room but distant	0.48 (1.18)	2.49* (6.77)	t'(53) = 2.027 (1 month)
	0.86 (1.67)	4.21* (7.44)	t'(40) = 2.544 (3 months)
Mother:			
Look at infant	85.89 (8.85)	67.36** (27.69)	t'(33) = 3.145 (6 months)
Smile at infant	12.64 (11.89)	6.18* (7.16)	F (1,34) = 4.17 (12 months)
	12 (13.3)	5.25* (6.5)	t'(27) = 2.066 (18 months)
No interactive behavior	14.11 (8.85)	24.92* (20.68)	t'(37) = 2.322 (6 months)
Infant:			
No interactive behavior	43.44 (12)	52* (12.6)	F (1,34) = 4.09 (12 months)

[a]
N @ 1 month: Rooming-in = 29, Control = 49; @ 3 months Rooming-in = 18, Control = 35;
@ 6 months Rooming-in = 15, Control = 26; @ 12 months Rooming-in = 14, Control = 22;
@ 18 months rooming-in = 20, Control = 23

[b]
Numbers are percentages of observed time with standard deviations in parentheses.

[c]
Infant age at which difference occurred   *p < .05   **p < .01

fant to none). Rooming-in mothers were more likely to continue signaling in isolation without infant response (mother to mother). Control dyads were more likely to signal sequentially but in isolation without entering mutual interaction (mother to infant). At three months, control infants were more likely to continue signaling in isolation without maternal response (infant to infant), while rooming-in children were more likely to cease signaling when mothers did not respond (infant to none). At six months, control infants were more likely not to respond (mother to none), and control pairs were more likely to abruptly discontinue mutual interaction (both to none).

At 12 months, control mothers were more likely to cease responding to their children (both to infant). Rooming-in infants were more likely to respond contingently to their mothers (mother to both) and rooming-in dyads were more likely to continue coacting (both to both). At 18 months, rooming-in children were more likely to respond contingently to their mothers (mother to both), while control infants were more likely not to respond (mother to none).

At six and 12 months, low-risk control dyads spent more observed time mutually inactive [dyadic state = none; rooming-in = 9%, control = 17%,

Table 4

Probability of Response During Mother-Infant Interaction: Low-Risk Sample

	Rooming-in	Control	F (df)
Mother:			
Response stops:			
Both → Infant	.023	.056*	F (1,34) = 5.49 (12 months)[a]
No response:			
Infant → Infant	.323	.466*	F (1,51) = 6.4 (3 months)
Infant → None	.076	.145*	F (1,77) = 3.93 (1 month)
	.200	.112*	$\overline{F}$ (1,51) = 5.41 (3 months)
Infant:			
Response given:			
Mother → Both	.269	.212*	F (1,34) = 5.17 (12 months)
	.268	.197*	$\overline{F}$ (1,41) = 5.98 (18 months)
No response:			
Mother → Mother	.817	.772*	F (1,77) = 4.44 (1 month)
Mother → None	.051	.086*	F (1,36) = 4.85 (6 months)
	.044	.066*	$\overline{F}$ (1,41) = 4.46 (18 months)
Mutual Response:			
Continues:			
Both → Both	.797	.717*	F (1,34) = 5.79 (12 months)
Stops:			
Both → None	.012	.032*	F (1,36) = 5.8 (6 months)
Does not occur:			
Mother → Infant	.004	.009**	F (1,77) = 7.47 (1 month)

[a] Infant age at which difference occurred

*p < .05

**p < .01

F (1,36) = 5.32, p < 0.05 at six months; rooming-in = 8%, control = 17%, F (1,34) = 9.81, p < 0.01 at 12 months]. At 12 months, low-risk rooming-in pairs spent more time coacting [dyadic state = both; rooming-in = 51%, control = 36%, F (1,34) = 10.34, p < .01].

High-risk. High-risk rooming-in and control groups differed on only two response transitions. At 12 months, high-risk rooming-in mothers were more likely to respond contingently to their infants [infant to both, .280 vs. .179, F (1,53) = 5.11, p < .05]. At 18 months, high-risk control infants were more likely not to respond to their mothers [mother to none, .055 vs. .036, F (1,44) = 5.79, p < .05].

Child Development

At nine months low-risk rooming-in and control infants did not differ in mental or motor development on the Bayley Scales. High-risk rooming-in children, however, were more advanced than high-risk control children in motor development on these scales at nine months [N: rooming-in = 15, control = 37; 112.33 ± 15.8 vs. 101.03 ± 16.8, F (1,50) = 4.99, p < 0.05].

Discussion

Because findings from earlier studies indicated that reduced parenting inadequacy following rooming-in apparently was due to an intermediary influence upon mother-infant interaction (O'Connor et al., 1980; O'Connor et al., Notes 1–3), it was anticipated that difference in interaction following rooming-in might be more prominent among that population of women at higher risk for child maltreatment than among low-risk women. Results from interaction observation do not indicate that this is the case. From one to 18 months postpartum (Table 3), high-risk rooming-in and control subjects differed significantly on only three of 115 comparisons made, less than the number of significant differences which might be found by chance. At 12 and 18 months, high-risk control mothers were more distant from their children, in the same room but not within arm's reach, while at 18 months, high-risk rooming-in mothers held their children more. In contrast to the minimal effects found within the high-risk group, results following rooming-in in the low-risk group resemble the pattern of findings of a previous report for a random sample of subjects (O'Connor et al., Notes 1, 2). This pattern suggests that rooming-in initially influences the context of mother-infant interactions and that this is followed in turn by expanding content of maternal and infant behaviors exchanged. In this report, at one and three months, low-risk rooming-in and control mother-infant interactions differed significantly in contextual factors of infant state and mother's proximity to her child and not in content of behaviors expressed. By six months, differences in the maternal behaviors of looking at and amount of time spent interacting with the child began to appear; and significant differences at 12 and 18 months involved only the content of interaction: mother smiling at her child and total amount of time the infant spent interacting with mother.

Results from the analyses of response transition probabilities emphasize the paucity of effects upon high-risk mother-infant interaction following rooming-in. High-risk dyadic interaction of rooming-in and control subjects differed in responsivity only twice. At 12 months, high-risk rooming-in mothers were more likely to join their infants in interaction (infant to both), and at 18 months, high-risk control mothers were more likely to cease signaling when their children failed to respond (mother to none). Within the low-risk group, however, the rooming-in and control groups differed on 12 of 60 comparisons of response transition probabilities. All but two of these significantly different comparisons were in the expected direction of increased responsivity of mother-infant interactions in the rooming-in group. The primary unexpected result occurred at three months when rooming-in mothers were more likely not to respond (infant to neither). This difference also appeared in an earlier report (O'Connor et al., Note 2) of a random sample testing consequences of rooming-in. For unclear reasons, all such contradictory differences between rooming-in and control in these investigations have occurred at three months (O'Connor et al., Note 1). The other difference found which might be considered unexpected occurred at one month when rooming-in infants were more likely not to respond (mother to mother). This result appeared only at one month, however, and it seems probable that this response transition, mother to mother, is more reflective of maternal pursuit of infant engagement rather than failure of response from the immature infant who was noted above to be less attentive due to drowsiness at one month.

In an earlier report involving a random sample (O'Connor et al., Note 3), it appeared that differences found between rooming-in and control groups during observation at 48 hours postpartum reflected only the different situational circumstances of rooming-in versus control experiences. This also appears to be true here. All of the differences between rooming-in and control groups at 48 hours (Table 2) might be expected. Rooming-in allowed more continuously satiated infants due to ad lib feeding, and therefore they could be expected to sleep more during observation. Rooming-in mothers had more flexible infant caretaking schedules and more time to examine their newborns. Control mothers, however, saw their infants only every four hours for feedings, so it is not surprising that during an observation held at feeding time control mothers did less nonfeeding caretaking, held their newborns more, and touched and looked at them more. These findings differ from results of studies in which the experimental variable was not extended contact but early mother-infant contact during the first three hours after delivery, where differences have been found at 36 to 96 hours suggestive of increased maternal involvement with the newborn following early mother-infant contact (Hales, Lozoff, Sosa, & Kennell, 1977; de Chateau & Winberg, 1977; Carlsson, Fogerberg, Horneman, Hwang, Larsson, Rodholm, Schaller, Danielsson, & Gundewall, 1978; Hittelman, Parekh, & Zilka, 1980; Lipper & Anisfeld, 1980). The lack of such differences in this study of extended contact without early contact suggests that early and extended contact may have different mechanisms of influencing the mother-child relationship.

In contrast to the unremarkable effects of rooming-in upon high-risk mother-infant interaction is the observation that high-risk rooming-in children scored significantly better in motor development at nine months than high-risk controls; low-risk rooming-in and control children did not differ developmentally. It appears then that outcome following rooming-in may vary depending upon measures used. If the measure is child development, as in this study, or adequacy in parenting, as in an earlier study (O'Connor et al., 1980), high-risk mothers and their infants will fare better. If, as in this study, the measure is mother-infant interaction, low-risk mother-infant dyads will appear most influenced by extended contact together. This results in a theoretical dilemma, however: how does rooming-in affect child development and parenting adequacy if not through an influence upon routine mother-infant interaction?

We believe that the influence of rooming-in parenting adequacy and child development within the high-risk group, in fact, is mediated through effects upon mother-infant interactions and that the interaction results within the low-risk group reflect, in an exaggerated manner, high-risk mother-infant interaction after rooming-in. It appears from the results for the low-risk group that rooming-in first facilitates early mother-infant adaptation, reflected in these data as the contectual differences between rooming-in and control at one and three months. Once this early mutual regulation has been established, it serves as an organizational framework within which an increasingly elaborate content of reciprocal behavioral exchange develops between mothers and infants who experienced rooming-in. This is reflected in these data by several significant behavioral results: rooming-in mothers looking at and interacting with their infants more at six months; rooming-in mothers and infants spending less observed time mutually inactive at six and 12 months and spending more time mutually interacting at 12 months; rooming-in mothers smiling at their infants more at 12 and 18 months; rooming-in children spending more time interacting with their mothers at 12 months; and the evidence provided in Table 4 for increased contingent responsivity during rooming-in mother-infant interaction. This serial effect of rooming-in upon mother-infant interaction could result in positive reinforcement of pleasurable mother-infant exchange and thereby explain how rooming-in might enhance longterm quality of parenting as has been found in other studies (Klaus et al., 1972; Kennell et al., 1974; Ringler et al., 1975; O'Connor et al., 1980).

The observational technology used in this investigation may have failed to detect this intermediary link between rooming-in and parenting/child development outcome in the high-risk group for several possible reasons. First, there were more multiparous women in the high-risk group than were in the low-risk group because the interview used to define risk prenatally favors primiparous women by giving them less opportunity to score negatively (Altemeier et al., 1979). As a consequence, there may have been more children present during interaction observation in high-risk homes to distract the mother from interacting with the younger child. In this case the findings for high-risk dyads might have resulted from a methodological artifact. The second possibility is that high-risk mothers were more inhibited by the observer than were low-risk mothers. Compared to the low-risk group, more high-risk mothers could be expected to have been under surveillance by authorities or neighbors for aberrant parenting, and this might have sensitized these mothers to observation by a stranger. Further, an interaction observation tends to be a bizarre social experience for mothers since an observing stranger is present whom they have been asked to ignore. High-risk mothers who have difficulty with any adult social exchange might find an interaction observation especially intimidating. Inhibition of high-risk mothers would explain why the only significant differences in duration of behaviors between high-risk rooming-in and control groups were those for mother's proximity to her child; high-risk mothers influenced by rooming-in but inhibited by an observer might be expected to remain physically closer to their children but otherwise quiescent. Information is available to support this possibility, since observer influence upon maternal behavior was evaluated after each interaction observation by a rating scale completed by the observer. Comparison of all high-risk versus all low-risk mothers at six months postpartum revealed that the high-risk mothers had been affected by the observer's presence [F (1,165) = 9.22, p < .01], and six months was the time when there were not even suggestive differences in high-risk rooming-in and control mother-infant interaction. High-risk and low-risk mothers did not differ on this rating scale, however, at other observation points. Both of these factors, in fact, may have contributed to the findings but, pending further research, any explanations for the apparent dichotomy between the effects of rooming-in upon mother-infant interaction versus development and parenting adequacy within the high-risk group remain speculative. It may be concluded, however, that findings in extra mother-infant postpartum contact research will vary with maternal risk status, measures employed for evaluation, and timing of the extra contact during the postpartum period.

REFERENCE NOTES

1. O'Connor, S., Vietze, P. M., Altemeier, W. A., Sandler, H. M., Sherrod, K. B., Falsey, S., Gerrity, S., & Hopkins, J. *Extended postpartum contact: I. Observation of maternal-infant interaction over the first year following rooming-in.* Manuscript submitted for publication, 1981.

2. O'Connor, S., Vietze, P. M., Sherrod, K. B., Sandler, H. M., Gerrity, S., Hopkins, J., & Altemeier, W. A. *Extended postpartum contact: II. Responsivity of maternal-infant interaction following rooming-in.* Manuscript submitted for publication, 1981.

3. O'Connor, S., Vietze, P. M., Sandler, H. M., Sherrod, K. B., Gerrity, S., Hopkins, J., & Altemeier, W. A. *Extended postpartum contact: III. Maternal and infant behavior during rooming-in.* Manuscript submitted for publication, 1981.

REFERENCES

Altemeier, W. A., Vietze, P. M., Sherrod, K. B., Sandler, H. M., Falsey, S., & O'Connor, S. Prediction of child maltreatment during pregnancy. *Journal of the American Academy of Child Psychiatry*, 1979, *18*, 205-218.

Altemeier, W. A., Vietze, P. M., Sherrod, K. B., Sandler, H. M., Tucker, D. D., & O'Connor, S. M. Prediction of child maltreatment in pregnancy. In S. Harel (Ed.), *The at risk infant*. Amsterdam: Excerpta Medica, 1980.

Anderson, B., Vietze, P. M., Faulstich, G., & Ashe, M. L. Observation manual for assessment of behavior sequences between infant and mother; Newborn to 24 months. *JSAS Catalog of Selected Documents*, 1978, *8*, 31.

Bakeman, R., & Brown, J. Behavioral dialogues: An approach to the assessment of mother-infant interaction. *Child Development*, 1977, *48*, 195-203.

Carlsson, F. G., Fagerberg, H., Horneman, G., Hwang, C. P., Larsson, K., Rodholm, M., Schaller, J., Danielsson, B., & Gundewall, C. Effects of amount of contact between mother and child on the mother's nursing behavior. *Developmental Psychology*, 1978, *11*, 143-150.

Cohler, B., Weiss, J., & Grunebaum, H. Childcare attitudes and emotional disturbance among mothers of young children. *Genetic Psychology Monographs*, 1970, *82*, 3-47.

DeChateau, P., & Winberg, B. Long-term effect on mother-infant behavior of the extra contact during the first hour postpartum. I. First observations at 36 hours. *Acta Paediatrica Scandinavia*, 1977, *66*, 137-144.

Hales, D. J., Lozoff, B., Sosa, R., & Kennell, J. H. Defining the limits of the maternal sensitive period. *Developmental Medicine and Child Neurology*, 1977, *19*, 454–461.

Hittelman, J., Parekh, A., Zilkha, S. Enhancing the birth experience: Assessing the effectiveness of the Laboyer method of child birth and early mother-infant contact. *Pediatric Research*, 1980, *14*, 434 (Abstract #52).

Holmes, T., & Rahe, R. The social readjustment rating scale. *Journal of Psychosomatic Research*, 1967, *11*, 213–218.

Kennell, J. H., Jerauld, R., Wolfe, H., Chesler, D., Kreger, N. C., McAlpine, W., Steffa, M., & Klaus, M. H. Maternal behavior one year after early and extended post-partum contact. *Developmental Medicine and Child Neurology*, 1974, *16*, 172–179.

Klaus, M. H., Jerauld, R., Kreger, N., McAlpine, W., Steffa, M., & Kennell, J. H. Maternal attachment: Importance of the first post-partum days. *New England Journal of Medicine*, 1972, *286*, 460–463.

Lewis, M., & Lee-Painter, S. An interactional approach to the mother-infant dyad. In M. Lewis & L. A. Rosenblum (Eds), *The effect of the infant on its caregiver*. New York: John Wiley & Sons, 1974.

Lipper, E. G., & Anisfeld, E. M. Effects of perinatal events on maternal-infant interaction. *Pediatric Research*, 1980, *14*, 435 (Abstract #57).

Myers, J. L. *Fundamentals of experimental design*. Boston: Allyn & Bacon, 1972, p. 73.

O'Connor, S., Vietze, P. M., Sherrod, K. B., Sandler, H. M., & Altemeier, W. A. Reduced incidence of parenting inadequacy following rooming-in. *Pediatrics*, 1980, *66*, 176–182.

O'Connor, S., Altemeier, W. A. Gerrity, S., Sandler, H. M., & Sherrod, K. A. Mother-infant interaction before ID of abuse, neglect or nonorganic failure-to-thrive. *Pediatric Research*, 1981, *15*, 454 (Abstract #85).

Ringler, N. M., Kennell, J. H., Jarvella, R., Navojosky, B. J., & Klaus, M. H. Mother-to-child speech at 2 years: Effects of early postnatal contact. *Journal of Pediatrics*, 1975, *86*, 141–144.

Siegel, E., Bauman, K. E., Schaefer, E. S., Saunders, M. M., & Ingram, D. D. Hospital and home support during infancy: Impact upon maternal attachment, child abuse and neglect, and health care utilization. *Pediatrics*, 1980, *66*, 183–190.

Vietze, P. M., Falsey, S., O'Connor, S., Sandler, H., Sherrod, K., & Altemeier, W. A. Newborn behavioral and interactional characteristics of nonorganic failure-to-thrive infants. In T. M. Field, S. Goldberg, D. Stern, & A. M. Sostek (Eds), *High risk infants and children*: *Adult and peer interactions*. New York: Academic Press, 1980.

Welch, B. L. The significance of the difference between two populations when the population variances are unequal. *Biometrika*, 1937, *29*, 350–362.

PSYCHOSOCIAL CHANGE IN RISK GROUPS: IMPLICATIONS FOR EARLY IDENTIFICATION

Richard Q. Bell
David Pearl

ABSTRACT. A consideration of psychosocial change in groups of infants and children at risk for schizophrenia, developmental retardation, delinquency, learning disability, substance abuse, child abuse, and hyperactivity leads to the conclusion that individuals are likely to move in and out of risk status as far as any given developmental phase is concerned. The frequency of review needed for disorders involving a long time span and major phases of development makes periodic developmental assessment by service providers more feasible than screening by an external screening team.

By forming risk groups in which development can be studied directly, it has been possible to move beyond retrospective reconstructions of etiology in several behavior disorders such as schizophrenia, developmental retardation, delinquency, and learning disability. The risk group approach is being expanded rapidly to many other areas of psychopathology on the basis of results from its application to the foregoing disorders. Though applications have been less extensive in other areas, there have been at least some successful efforts to apply the approach to substance abuse and child abuse. In addition, there is a prospect of its application to hyperactivity.

One of the problems of identifying a risk group, the possibility of a self-fulfilling prophecy, appears to be less serious than originally thought, whereas a new problem has emerged, the fact that children move in and out of risk as developmental and contextual factors in their lives change. These changes imply the need for a more frequent, more developmentally and ecologically oriented screening. Who can perform such screening for the many phases of growth in infancy and childhood? This paper will review problems and possible solutions to the problems of transactional risk, against the background of findings in the foregoing seven areas of research.

Richard Q. Bell is Chief, Behavioral Sciences Research Branch, National Institute of Mental Health, Room 10C09, Parklawn Building, 5600 Fishers Lane, Rockville, MD 20857. Reprints may be obtained from Richard Q. Bell, Psychology Department, Gilmer Hall, University of Virginia, Charlottesville, VA 22901.

David Pearl is at the National Institute of Mental Health, Adelphi, MD.

The Concept of Risk

As used in this paper, the concept of risk implies the ability to identify groups of individuals who, on the average, do not now show a disorder, or only show components of the disorder, but who have a statistically significant likelihood of showing the disorder in full form at a later time, in comparison with a non-risk group. It is not necessary that the level of efficiency in prediction be so great as to make the prediction of the outcome possible for individuals. The concept applies to a group. It is accepted that many individuals in the group may never show the later disorder, even though the group as a whole shows a significant elevation of risk. Although the concept has a long history of usage in medicine, it was introduced to the field of behavior pathology by Mednick and McNeil (1968) in order to escape the stalemate of reliance on retrospective reconstructions from clinical groups that are subject to unknown sampling bias, or the immense difficulty of marshalling large-scale and long-term collaborative studies that would be necessary to follow an unselected group of children for 25 years in order to obtain a 1% sub-sample of schizophrenics.

Examples of Risk Research

Schizophrenia. This behavioral disorder has received considerable attention and involved international collaboration. Children at risk for schizophrenia can be identified on the basis of a schizophrenic spectrum disorder in one parent. It is only necessary to work from hospital or other community records to locate schizophrenic adults, then further screen for those that are married and have children. A large source population is necessary as is full cooperation of community institutions and agencies that have jurisdiction over records and offer a means of locating individuals at risk.

Since it is possible to establish a group at considerably greater risk for schizophrenia than the usual expectation of 1% (the incidence being 10% for children with one schizophrenic parent), and since risk can be determined for infants or children selected at any of the periods along the developmental course, age segments of the disorder can be studied in different samples. Hopefully, the developmental pathway leading to a schizophrenic spectrum disorder in the child can be reconstructed, segment by segment, each segment studied simultaneously or nearly so, and even by different research groups, greatly accelerating the progress toward understanding the etiology (Garmezy, 1974). The studies of age segments may even be articulated, as is being attempted in a University of Rochester study (Wynne, 1981) following what has been termed a convergent or accelerated longitudinal approach (Bell, 1953). Three separate groups of risk children were initially studied at ages 4, 7, and 10, then were followed up at ages 7, 10, and 13 with similar measures at comparable initial and follow-up assessment, so that the age 7 follow-up measurement of the age 4 group can be compared with the initial measurement of the age 7 group, and so on.

Whether or not the latter refinements in approach are possible, the important fact is that direct developmental study of the disorder can be pursued in any of the age ranges desired. Of course, we do not know yet whether these research results can be applied to the 90% of the schizophrenic population that does not have one schizophrenic parent (but may have schizophrenic relatives). Yet we can at least say that, for a subgroup, in heredity there is hope. Due to the genetic contribution, the continuity in one variant of the disorder can be studied despite different age manifestations. There is the possibility of more rapid research progress based on data from direct study of the course of the disorder as it unfolds, rather than from inferences and extrapolations based on late forms of the illness. Progress in the prospective study of the disorder provides the hope, in turn, for more effective early identification and intervention, based on a more complete knowledge of the actual course. Furthermore, evidence mentioned later in this paper indicates that the fact of a genetic or congenital contributor in no sense implies immutability. The existence of risk lasting for many years does not imply that the emergence of pathology is inevitable.

Developmental retardation. Severe complications of pregnancy or delivery constitute a well established basis for risk (see Werner, Bierman, & French, 1971, for a review). The sub-group that has been studied most intensively is low birth weight infants born before the expected date of delivery. It is only necessary to work from medical records to establish the existence of risk for adverse development. If the necessary information is in the records, the risk may be established in the neonatal period, in later infancy, childhood, or even adulthood. Although an extensive literature establishing the existence of risk has been built up, risk and non-risk groups overlap greatly on most behavior measures, and differences narrow so much by the second year of life that a treatment program is not appropriate unless prematurity is associated with other conditions. Findings from the Kauai study (Werner et al., 1971) indicate that the interaction of severe complications of pregnancy or delivery (of which low birth weight is one) with low SES, family instability, and low maternal intelligence, established a group at risk of developmental retardation up to age two years. This interaction is overshadowed at age ten by family background factors such as low SES, lack of educational stimulation, and lack of emotional support. The effects of complications of pregnancy and delivery as such were still detectable at that age but were attenuated.

Many of the Head Start research projects selected children at risk of developmental retardation on the basis of low SES level alone (Bronfenbrenner, 1975). However, one of the projects that showed the most clear evidence of initial risk in the contrast groups (Heber & Garber, 1975) selected infants from families living in census tracts known to have residents primarily living in poverty, then further screened for those whose mothers had a measured IQ at or below 75.

Anti-social behavior. The determination of risk for delinquency, aggressive behavior, and other anti-social problems has been pursued actively for decades. Only a few of the numerous longitudinal studies have defined their risk groups in advance. Lundman and Scarpitti (1978) and West and Farrington (1973) review this research, and the latter report their own findings from a study that was actually predictive, though some risk groups were formed after the completion of the study from data that would have been available at the outset. Out of a sample of 411 eight- and nine-year-old males located in six schools serving a crowded working class area in which public housing predominated, various risk groups ranging from 55 to 95 in size were formed. Each risk group was formed based on different criteria. Then the risk groups were compared with the rest of the sample on number of convictions up to age 17.

Although details on false positives and negatives involved in predicting each of the seven disorders would encumber this manuscript unduly, data will be furnished for this one study to illustrate the problems of prediction that are typical for many other behavior disorders, and to provide a basis for an observation on phases of risk research in which errors of prediction are or are not critical. Returning to the study by West and Farrington (1973), early background factors such as low family income, large family, criminality in the parents, and inadequate parental guidance, predicted later convictions just as well as did measures of incipient delinquency (e.g., ratings of conduct disorder and troublesomeness in the child). However, less than half of the risk children actually became delinquent, and most of the future delinquents were not in the risk groups. In the risk group based on background factors, the correct labelling of 31 future delinquents was achieved at the expense of incorrectly labelling 32, and overlooking 53 delinquents. This level of prediction is below requirements for intervention programs that can rarely afford to treat twice as many children as need help, but is sufficient for research purposes if we merely wish to reconstruct conceptually the pathways by which children become delinquent.

In contrast with the early identification of infants or children at risk for schizophrenia or developmental retardation, the task of forming risk groups is much more difficult, requiring that information be obtained from juvenile authorities, schools, and families. Nonetheless, in the studies that the foregoing authors reviewed, it has already been amply demonstrated that this task is feasible in a variety of communities and in different countries. The task of designing interventions that will have sustained long-range effects, on the other hand, has proved to be extremely difficult.

Learning disability. Risk studies have been carried out on learning disability as an overall category as well as one of its major component problems, dyslexia. A study by Keogh, Welles, and Hall (1976) reported that overall ratings of risk by kindergarten teachers, as well as ratings of reading readiness, ability to pay attention, follow directions, and ability to get along with other children, predicted learning disability in the first through second grades. Silver, Hagin, and Beecher (1978) have approached the problem of identifying kindergarten and early school-age children at risk of developing dyslexia by employing a rapid screening test. This test is based on the assessment of delayed development in visual, auditory and body image perception presumed to mediate the reading process. Satz and Friel (1978) have also developed a test battery to detect children at risk of dyslexia. This battery involves several verbal and non-verbal perceptual tests. In a longitudinal study starting with kindergarten children they have been successful in predicting both successful and unsuccessful readers. As in the case of the other studies of learning disability, Satz's goal was early detection of risk in order to make possible timely preventive or remedial treatment of the child at risk. Such early intervention is seen as forestalling or minimizing the serious secondary emotional and behavioral problems which can arise from a child's sense of academic failure, a negative self-concept, and overall frustration.

Substance abuse. The empirical base for early identification of risk groups is just beginning to accrue in two other disorders. One of the most promising areas for both screening and possible intervention is that of substance abuse (e.g., marijuana, cocaine, heroin). A weighted composite of grades, peer ratings of obedience, and child self-reports of rebelliousness, cigarette smoking and attitudes toward smoking, all obtained in the seventh to eighth grades, was used to identify users versus non-users two years later (Smith & Fogg, 1979).

Child abuse. Public interest in child abuse is high. The base for determination of risk for abuse is just emerging. The fact that a clearly predictive study of risk has appeared early in the development of this relatively new area of research, may indicate increasing recognition of the utility of the risk approach, in addition to the impetus coming from extensive research on mother-infant bonding in maternity hospitals (Klaus & Kennell, 1976). A report by Gray, Cutler, Dean, and Kempe (1979) indicates a small number of cases of child abuse in a group of 50 mothers selected during labor and delivery as at risk of abnormal parenting, on the basis of lack of interest in the baby. No cases of abuse occurred in a similar group receiving supportive intervention, or in another group of 50 not showing any signs of risk. From the efforts of professional and lay leaders to draw public attention to child abuse, it has become increasingly evident that there are more cases in the general population than previously expected. However, this is still a low base-rate disorder, and thus the fact that only a small number of cases emerged in the risk-without-intervention group should not be taken as an indication that this study is only working with a weak relationship. Much larger numbers of subjects are needed in future studies which, it is hoped, will develop out of this first effort.

Hyperactivity. Only the possibility of forming a risk group exists at present for disorders involving inability to sustain attention, frequent changes in goal direction, and inadequate control over impulses. There have been several longitudinal and many retrospective studies but these have been concerned with the later childhood and adult fate of the hyperactive, not with the detection of prior risk.

Two recent studies may open up the possibility that a risk group can be identified. Waldrop, Bell, McLaughlin, and Halverson (1978) reported a high level of prediction in a sample of males originally given a brief ten-minute examination in the newborn period for minor physical anomalies. These children were then followed up to the early preschool period, when they were studied intensively for a month. The number of anomalies predicted whether the individual showed fast-moving, impulsive, and distractible play at the preschool period. From continuity studies, it has been shown that the brief examination could be given at any time from the newborn period through the early school-age years with equal validity.

A more recent study (Schexnider, Bell, Shebilske, & Quinn, 1981) has shown that an attention deficit can be demonstrated as early as the first year of infancy in males who have a large number of minor physical anomalies. The latter group habituates more rapidly when fatigued, more slowly when fresh, in comparison with a group showing a small number of anomalies. Thus, it seems possible to form a risk group prior to the emergence of hyperactivity, based on both the count of anomalies and the attentional deficit. In contrast with the positive results from these studies, only low order prediction was found in a sample studied only briefly at follow-up (Burg, Hart, Quinn, & Rappoport, 1978), but this result may have been due to lack of behavior aggregation, as described by Epstein (1980).

Labeling

The establishment of risk groups involves the potential problem of negative labeling. Whenever a presumed unfavorable outcome has been assigned to a group, the possibility exists that this fact will be communicated to those who are directly interacting with or making decisions about the management of members of that group. Resulting changes in social feedback may then lock the member of the risk group into deviant status. The maintenance of a deviant role can then become part of the socialization process for individuals affected. However, negative labeling does not explain the development of deviance. Nor can it be assumed that labeling a child or family is "at risk" in the files of an investigator or service program will in itself have adverse consequences unless there is a reasonable basis for specifying the process by which it will occur. A review of the literature on labeling and substance abuse (Williams, 1976) is particularly relevant to the areas of risk with which this paper is concerned.

Delinquency is an area similar to substance abuse in sensitivity to problems of negative labeling. Williams' review indicates that there is a complex relationship between the labeling agent, the individual's reference group, and self-concept. The research evidence is far short of supporting the existence of any infallible process that automatically ensues once labeling has occurred. An example of the complexity of this issue was cited by Williams. Thirty-nine percent of a sample of blind children answered a direct question by saying that they did not consider themselves blind. From this and many other examples in Williams' review it is very evident that blanket statements about the likelihood of labeling occurring cannot be made. Relationships between key elements in the process of labeling are quite variable. Each research and service program must be evaluated individually against the likelihood of adverse affects. However, it is reassuring that for over fifteen years research has been carried out in an extremely sensitive risk area, schizophrenia, without any evidence of adverse consequences to members of this risk group. At the same time, considerable experience has accumulated amongst the staffs of these projects in protecting subjects against labeling effects, experience that is available to others in the field by informal contacts.

Issues in Early Identification and Screening

Screening without Service

A recent review of a successful screening program in Sweden (Wagner, 1975) has recommended that screening be limited to conditions that can be treated, and for which service providers are available. These recommendations have the obvious purpose of avoiding expensive and fruitless screening that alarms families and then leaves them frustrated in efforts to get help. However, the objectives of screening for research on risk groups differ from those for provision of services, to which the foregoing report refers. First of all, to check the validity of risk criteria, it will frequently be necessary to identify groups for which no treatment is currently available. For example, there is no existing treatment program for one-year-old infants at risk of later hyperactivity because of minor physical anomalies and attentional deficits. The purpose of screening at an early stage of research on a risk group is to determine whether the presumed risk group actually differs on important behaviors at home, or in the community setting, in at least one important phase of development. The next step is to determine whether screening in other phases also reveals meaningful differences. If characteristic behaviors revealed in different phases of development make it possible to reconstruct the course of development, an optimal point and method of intervention may become evident. At that point, research comparing various methods of intervention is appropriate and, finally, the reservations expressed by Wagner (1975) become relevant concerning availability of a mode of treatment and service providers. For the foregoing reasons, it is inadvisable to suspend screening for research until such elements are available.

In contrast to the problems of establishing risk for hyperactivity, a mode of intervention and an optimal time were available to the investigators of child abuse, coming from a large number of studies on bonding (Klaus & Kennell, 1976). This application illustrates the extent to which screening and intervention in risk programs are dependent on the fund of knowledge developed in the general field of early development.

Early Identification Based on Changing Risk Status

If we see the members of a risk group as having fixed risk status, then our task is to identify them prior to a period in which intervention is most efficacious. This approach follows the medical model of early diagnosis followed by an appropriate treatment program. However, it is inappropriate to risk groups subject to psychosocial change, as Beckman-Brindley and Bell (1981) have pointed out. If, in keeping with Sameroff's thesis (1977), we see risk as a transaction between the individual and the environment, rather than as a property of the individual, it should not be surprising that individuals move in and out of risk status. Even in the case of physical disabilities in which a congenital contribution is strong, such transactions are critical to determining whether a child is at risk during a given period. A child with an established risk due to cerebral palsy may have great difficulty with peers in the neighborhood, but later function adequately with no behavior disorder in a special nursery school in which other children have been taught how to react to the limitations imposed by the disorder.

The nature of the school to which a child is sent (Rutter, 1979) or, as in the case of risk for substance abuse, the nature of the particular peer groups to which the child is exposed (Kandel, 1980) may determine whether behavior pathology emerges. A child who apparently is functioning well in one period, subsequently may show behavior pathology after exposure to a noxious interpersonal setting. Many middle-class parents, who have felt they did well as parents and have provided many advantages in education and material support for their children, have been quite surprised to find their children heavily involved in substance abuse and illegal sales.

The concept of long-term jeopardy overriding many years or major developmental phases is only applicable to risk groups such as (1) the genetically linked sub-group of individuals at risk of schizophrenia, (2) individuals congenitally at risk for hyperactivity, and (3) the physically handicapped. We have cited examples from this latter category, although it has not been elaborated as a risk category because it is customarily treated separately from the behavior disorders. Even in the foregoing categories, just as in substance abuse and delinquency, individuals may not actually show behavior pathology during any given period, nor even ultimately manifest the condition which was the basis for setting up the risk group. In contrast with the foregoing categories, an initial determination of risk is sufficient in the case of child abuse, reading and attention disorders. The interval to determination of outcome for the risk studies cited is only 17 months in the former, one school year in the case of the latter.

The selection of phases of development in which periodic reviews take place should be based largely on the salient features and key processes known to be underway during the age range. For example, based on a research summary by Emde, Gaensbauer, and Harmon (1976), one review might be set at the end of the second month to determine which mothers are showing appropriate attachment to their infants and to determine which infants have shown the expected reduction of fussing and crying which might otherwise stress the mother-infant relationship (Bell, 1977, p. 135). The next review might be at the end of seven months to determine whether the infant is manifesting a social smile and behaving discriminately toward adults (and also to determine which mothers are responsive to the new social stimuli provided by the infant). Subsequent reviews might occur at the end of the first year or 18 months, when the attachment mechanism of infant to mother and vice versa could be more completely evaluated.

Developmental Review by Service Providers

The outlook for quick screening for a variety of childhood behavior disorders in large populations of infants and children is bleak (Children's Defense Fund, 1977; American Association of Psychiatric Services for Children, 1977) because of the lack of brief screening instruments and the complexities of assessing individuals who are changing rapidly with development, and whose conditions cannot be considered apart from their context. For example, a moderately retarded child may function adequately in the family and neighborhood of an ethnic group that finds roles and functions for its handicapped, but pose serious problems in a neighborhood of much more affluent but isolated families who interact with each other very little and expect each family to take care of its own problems. However, the bleak outlook may in part be due to the fact that we are looking in the wrong direction for first line screening. Such screening is going on all the time informally by individuals who are in contact with infants and young children. Bower (1977) has made an excellent case for having developmental review carried out by service providers. First of all, service providers such as day care, nursery, and elementary school teachers have a much better observation base for making statements about a child than any quick assessment could provide. They see the individual functioning in at least one important context and have the advantage of being able to aggregate behaviors over time, a critical factor in overcoming instability of measurement in the social and behavioral sciences, as Epstein (1980) has pointed out.

Teachers' judgments are surprisingly accurate in predicting learning disablity, though Satz and Friel (1978) note that teachers predicted severe reading disability less efficiently than the tests because of concern over labeling effects. Also, the study by Keogh, Welles, and Hall (1976), already cited as an example of how risk for learning disability can be established, indicates that screening for learning disability may be carried out be service providers. They found that teachers' ratings of risk and its components predicted later learning disability in the first through second grades better than the objective tests used. It is surprising that heterogeneous ratings from several schools and many teachers were so effective. One interpretation of their results (Hall, Note 1) provides a basis for also expecting that developmental review by service providers may, in some cases, be more useful than any quick screening system, except for special perceptual or motor problems and sensory handicaps requiring instrument technology for screening. The teachers' judgments were made in the context of the classroom placements and school systems to which their children would be exposed, a type of accommodation to the child's own criterion situation that an objective test could not reflect. This judgment of the criterion situation, which varies so greatly from one school to the next, could prove more important than the lower objectivity and uniformity inherent in ratings. Accordingly, in addition to the fact that service providers have more extensive contact with infants and children than a screening team could have, judgments by the many different service providers in the family, peer, school, and community contexts to which the child will have to adjust, may be a vital part of the screening.

To say that service providers should carry out periodic developmental reviews means that day care center, nursery school, kindergarten, and primary school teachers should be relied upon for this function. Although the legal aspects of the Education for all Handicapped Children Act of 1975 (P.L. 94-142) have proved to be very burdensome to school administrators, its mandates have made it possible for most school systems to demonstrate that they can screen their school population and then provide a comprehensive developmental review for selected children with developmental retardation, and emotional and learning disorders. A less cumbersome and legalistic system could quite conceivably carry out the periodic reviews needed for most of the risk groups we have reviewed. Schools provide a comprehensive coverage of children from a community population. The problems of heterogeneity of standards for screening, fallibility of teachers' judgments, labeling, and many other problems of administering such programs immediately come to mind, but these can be solved by social and behavioral engineering skills already available to our field. Thus, these problems should not distract our attention from the basic information relevant to screening that is available to service providers.

What can be done about the period from pregnancy up to the child's entry into school? The mother passes through the facilities of such service providers as gynecologists, obstetricians and their nurses, prenatal clinics, and the pediatric personnel in newborn nurseries, hospitals, and well-baby clinics. After these contacts, however, many family units may not be reachable until the kindergarten period. Substantial numbers of the infant and child population are not placed in day care centers or nursery schools. In addition, as Rolf has pointed out in this same volume, many families, especially those whose members are at risk, do not utilize services and facilities available to them and, in fact, are often difficult for service providers to approach. Developmental review by service providers from the period of pregnancy forward to the time a child enters school would therefore require a restructuring and organization of community service providers, and possibly the provision of services where they do not now exist. Wagner's report (1975) summarizing Sweden's experience with early screening, to which we have already referred, indicates greatest success using parents and physicians to screen four-year-olds. He also concluded that screening should be limited to such clearly diagnosed problems as those involving vision, hearing, and physiological disorders. This may indeed by the case and we may have to turn to other possibilities for screening of behavior disorders.

The BEEP project in Boston (Pierson, Levine, & Wolman, 1981) provides one model of how screening and service can be combined in an urban school system for the entire period of early infancy and cover the behavior disorders as well as the more easily diagnosed conditions. In the case of this project, it was realized by school administrators that many of the problems faced by teachers and other school personnel in kindergarten and first grade could have been anticipated and corrected more easily if there had been access to these children much earlier in development. That is, cases of hyperactivity, developmental retardation, and learning disability had become "hardened" by the time they reach the school system, making rehabilitation efforts and intervention much more difficult and time consuming.

A disorder that goes on for several years produces circular negative feedback between parents and affected children and between those affected children and their siblings or peers. It is much more difficult to work with the mother of a kindergartener whose perceptions of the child's behavior have become quite negative and stabilized than with the same mother when she may have only begun to experience a somewhat unrewarding and difficult behavior pattern in the same child as an infant.

The BEEP project located expectant mothers, then offered a variety of services such as home visits and an open-house visiting center for them and their infants, in addition to behavior development and pediatric examinations. The sample of 285 infants was in frequent contact with staff who identified many medical and developmental problems during the age range 8–18 months, and assisted the parents or obtained referrals.

The key problem in periodic developmental review, then, is to organize and supplement community services so that the total cohort of infants or children can be assessed by individuals in frequent contact with them during important developmental phases. From the standpoint of disorders involving changing psychosocial risk, an age-specific total cohort review by service providers would be required. While this sounds as though it is an overwhelming task, and from the standpoint of community organization it may indeed prove to be very difficult, in many ways it may be much easier to accomplish than periodic mass screening by an external team. Infants or children require no special contact if they are not seen as currently having problems, or anticipated to have problems in the next developmental phase or setting.

In mass screening, by contrast, all cases have to be contacted and assessed. Furthermore, most mass screening requires successive screenings and filters to eliminate false positives (Frankenberg, Kemper, van Doorninck, Dick, & Fandal, Note 2). Essentially these multiple contacts are needed to offset inadequate information about the child at the outset. Daily or frequent contact by a service provider, however, produces such information routinely. It is probably easier to train and calibrate service providers, or devise some system to obtain screening information from them, than it is to bypass them and attempt to attain the same information base through screening by an external team.

Implications for Risk Research and Early Identification

A new perspective on risk research is emerging out of a transactional approach to development, one that considers the many developmental and contextual changes that occur over major developmental periods in the lives of children. The task of risk research for all but the disorders with a short incubation time will be to reconstruct, segment by segment, the developmental and contextual processes by which pathology develops. Once the pathways by which the disorder emerges become clear, an optimal time and mode of screening and intervention can be devised for each disorder. From this standpoint, early identification for the purpose of referring a child to an intervention program should seldom be based on results from a single contrast between risk and non-risk groups. Multiple contrasts will be needed.

In the case of disorders such as schizophrenia, delinquency, substance abuse, and hyperactivity, screening and re-screening will be needed at major developmental phases because children will move in and out of risk status as their transactions with their environment change. Frequent developmentally and contextually oriented screening will be needed. Periodic review should be set to capture risk-relevant aspects of salient features during major phases of development. This kind of screening activity, in turn, requires greater use of service providers in first line screening, whether in infant care centers, pediatric facilities, day-care centers, nursery or elementary schools. Individuals in these facilities are familiar with the developmental characteristics of the age range, and have far more contact with the children than any external screening team. Whether or not a risk condition is permanent (e.g., one parent with a schizophrenic spectrum disorder, a congenital contributor to hyperactivity, physical handicaps), age-specific developmental review will be needed to determine if the child is actually in need of referral during any given phase of development.

REFERENCE NOTES

1. Hall, R., Personal communication. This interpretation developed out of a discussion with Robert Hall and the present author. It should not be ascribed to the other authors of the report in question.
2. Frankenberg, W. K., Kemper, M., van Doorninck, W. J., Dick, N. P., & Fandal, A. *Validation of a three-stage developmental screening procedure.* Undated paper No. 211-24-9966, University of Colorado Medical Center, Denver, Colorado.

REFERENCES

American Association of Psychiatric Services for Children. *Developmental review in the early periodic screening, diagnosis and treatment program: Final report, 1977.* U. S. Dept. of HEW, HCFA, Medicaid Bureau (HCFA 77-29437.)

Beckman-Brindley, S., & Bell, R. Q. Issues in early identification. In J. M. Kaufman & D. P. Hallahan (Eds.), *Handbook of special education.* Englewood Cliffs, New Jersey: Prentice-Hall, 1981.

Bell, R. Q. An experimental test of the accelerated longitudinal approach. *Child Development,* 1953, *25* , 281–286.

Bell, R. Q., & Harper, L. V. *Child effects on adults.* Hillsdale, New Jersey: Lawrence Erlbaum Assoc., 1977.

Bower, E. M. Mythologies, realities, possibilities. In G. W. Albee & J. M. Joffe (Eds.), *Primary prevention of psychopathology, Vol. I: The issues.* Hanover, N.H.; University Press of New England, 1977.

Bronfenbrenner, U. Is early intervention effective. In B. Z. Friedlander, G. M. Sterritt, & G. E. Kirk (Eds.), *Exceptional infant, Vol. 3; Assessment and intervention.* New York: Brunner-Mazel, 1975. 449–475.

Burg, D., Hart, E., Quinn, P., & Rappoport, J. Newborn minor physical anomalies and prediction of infant behavior. *Journal of Autism & Childhood Schizophrenia,* 1978, *8,* 427–439.

Children's Defense Fund of the Washington Research Project, Inc. *EPSDT: Does it spell health care for poor children?* Washington, D.C.: Children's Defense Fund, 1977

Emde, R. N., Gaensbauer, T. J., & Harmon, R. J. Emotional expression in infancy: A biobehavioral study. *Psychological Issues, Monograph Series,* 1976, *10,* No. 1.

Epstein, S. The stability of behavior: II. Implications for psychological research. *American Psychologist,* 1980, *35,* 790–806.

Garmezy, N. Children at risk: The search for antecedents of schizophrenia. Part I. Conceptual models and research methods. *Schizophrenia Bulletin*, 1974, *8*, 14–90.

Gray, J., Cutler, C., Dean, J., & Kempe, C. H. Prediction and prevention of child abuse. *Seminars in Perinatology*, 1979, *3*, 85–90.

Heber, R., & Garber, H. The Milwaukee Project: A study of the use of family intervention to prevent cultural-familial mental retardation. In B. Z. Friedlander, G. M. Sterrit, & G. E. Kirk (Eds.), *Exceptional infant, Vol 3: Assessment and intervention*. New York: Brunner-Mazel, 1975.

Kandel, D. B. Drug and drinking behavior among youth. In A. Inkeles, J. Coleman, & R. H. Turner (Eds.), *Annual Review of Sociology*, 1980, *6*, 235–285.

Keogh, B. K., Welles, M. F., & Hall, R. J. An approach to early identification of high potential and high risk pupils. *Technical Report SERP 1976-Al*. Los Angeles: Graduate School of Education, University of California, 1976.

Klaus, M. H., & Kennell, J. H. *Maternal-infant bonding*. St. Louis, Missouri: C. V. Mosby, 1976.

Lundman, R. J., & Scarpitti, F. R. Delinquency prevention: recommendations for future research. *Crime & Delinquency*, 1978, *24*, 207–220.

Mednick, S. A., & McNeil, P. S. Current methodology in research the etiology of schizophrenia: Serious difficulties which suggest the use of the high risk approach. *Psychological Bulletin*, 1968, *70*, 681–693.

Pierson, D. E., Levine, M. D., & Wolman, R. Auditing multidisciplinary assessment procedures: A system developed for the Brookline Early Education Project. In W. K. Frankenburg & N. Anastasiow (Eds.), *Identifying the developmentally delayed child*. University Park, Maryland: University Park Press. In press, 1981.

Rutter, M. Protective factors in children's responses to stress and disadvantage. In M. W. Kent & J. E. Rolf (Eds.), *Primary prevention of psychopathology, Vol. III: Social competence in children*. Hanover, N.H.: University Press of New England, 1979.

Sameroff, A. J. Concepts of humanity. In G. W. Albee & J. M. Joffee (Eds.), *Primary prevention of psychopathology, Vol. I: The issues*. Hanover, N.H.: University Press of New England, 1977.

Satz, P., & Friel, J. Predictive validity of an abbreviated screening battery. *Journal of Learning Disabilities*. 1978, *6*, 347–351.

Schexnider, V. Y. R., Bell, R. Q., Shebilske, W. L., & Quinn, P. Habituation of visual attention in infants with minor physical anomalies. *Child Development*, in press, 1981.

Silver, A. A., Hagin, R. A., & Beecher, R. Scanning: Diagnosis and intervention in prevention of reading disability. Part I, Search: The scanning measure. *Journal of Learning Disabilities*, 1978, *11*, 434–445.

Smith, G. M., & Fogg, C. P. Psychological antecedents of teen-age drug use. In R. G. Simmons (Ed.), *Research in community and mental health* , Vol. 1. Greenwich, Connecticut: JAI Press, 1979.

Wagner, M. *Sweden's health-screening program for four-year old children*. National Institute of Mental Health, Rockville, Maryland, 1975.

Waldrop, M. F., Bell, R. Q., McLaughlin, B., & Halverson, C. Newborn minor physical anomalies predict short attention span, peer aggression and impulsivity at age 3. *Science*, 1978, *199*, 563–564.

Werner, E. E., Bierman, J. M., & French, E. E. *The Children of Kauai: A longitudinal study from the prenatal period to age ten*. Honolulu: University of Hawaii Press, 1971.

West, D. J., & Farrington, D. P. *Who becomes delinquent*. London: Heineman, 1973.

Williams, J. R. Effects of labeling the ''drug-abuser'': An inquiry. *National Institute on Drug Abuse Research Monograph*, 6, 1976.

Wynne, L. The University of Rochester child and family study: Overview of research plan. In N. Watt, E. J. Anthony, L. Wynne, & J. Rolf (Eds.), *Children at risk for schizophrenia: A longitudinal perspective*. New York: Cambridge University Press, in press, 1981.

PRIMARY PREVENTION
OF DEVELOPMENTAL RETARDATION
DURING INFANCY

Craig T. Ramey
Joseph J. Sparling
Donna M. Bryant
Barbara H. Wasik

ABSTRACT. This review examines eighteen exemplary prevention-oriented early intervention programs designed for high-risk and normal infants. The target populations, the form of the program delivery, and the content of the curriculum are described. Issues in the design and methodology of such programs are discussed. The review also summarizes continuing and delayed effects of early intervention programs with an emphasis on those projects that had a follow-up evaluation phase. Finally, three theoretical perspectives are presented. These perspectives have important implications for infant program planning and evaluation from which recommendations are made for future programs designed for high-risk infants.

The behavioral and health sciences have a long history of professional concern with developmental retardation. Since the time of Seguin and Itard (1932), educators and psychologists have sought to improve the intellectual and adaptive behavior of retarded children through systematic training regimens. Only recently, however, have there been programmatic efforts designed to *prevent* mild developmental retardation.

This relatively new, but growing, emphasis on prevention appears to be a by-product of several theoretical and social trends which have emerged over the past two decades in American child psychology and related services. Four trends are particularly noteworthy as major contributors to the prevention emphasis. First, beginning with Hunt's (1961) book, *Intelligence and Experience*, there has been a systematic appreciation of the potential power

This research was supported, in part, by the Bureau of Education for the Handicapped contract 300 77 0309/04 and the Administration for Children, Youth and Families grant 90 CW 602/02. Reprints may be obtained from Craig T. Ramey, Frank Porter Graham Child Development Center, University of North Carolina, Highway 54, Bypass West, Chapel Hill, NC 27514.

Joseph J. Sparling, Donna M. Bryant, and Barbara H. Wasik are affiliated with the University of North Carolina at Chapel Hill, Chapel Hill, NC.

of early experience to alter or modify at least some components of early intelligence. This realization has been spurred by the now vast number of empirical studies demonstrating the remarkable capacities of human infants to learn. Second, there has been a confluence of studies (Knoblock & Pasamanick, 1953; Golden, Birns, Bridges, & Moss, 1971; Ramey & Campbell, 1979) demonstrating that it is during the second year of life that differences in the cognitive abilities of children from different socioeconomic strata become apparent. These differences almost always favor children from the economically and socially advantaged segments of our society. The third trend is the human potential movement of the 1960s and 1970s. This movement created a social action climate in the United States which resulted in an unparalleled professional dedication to helping socially disadvantaged families participate more fully in the American educational and economic mainstream. The fourth noteworthy trend is the increasing emphasis on cost-benefit analysis that has prodded human service providers to seek efficient as well as effective means to aid the development of disadvantaged children and families.

These four major trends contributed to the creation of innovative child and family education programs targeted toward the socially disadvantaged. Reviews of some of these programs have been conducted by Stedman and his colleagues (Stedman, Anastasiow, Dokecki, Gordon, & Parker, Note 1), Bronfenbrenner (1975), Haskins, Finkelstein, and Stedman (1978), and the Lazar group (Darlington, Royce, Snipper, Murray, & Lazar, 1980). Some of these intervention programs began when the children were in infancy, but most began during the later preschool years of the child. A shift in emphasis to programs beginning in infancy occurred later, primarily as a result of the evaluation of Project Head Start that showed retardation was not being ameliorated (Westinghouse, 1969).

It is the purpose of this article to review exemplary prevention-oriented programs which began in the child's first two years of life. First the target populations, the form of the program delivery, and the content of the curriculum will be described. Then issues in the design and methodology of intervention programs will be discussed. Finally, concepts that have implications for creating a new generation of such programs will be identified and specific program features that need to be incorporated into the creation and evaluation of new preventive educational efforts will be suggested.

Target, Form and Content of Intervention Programs

From the mid 1960s to the 1980s, programs for early intervention have varied in the target of intervention, the form of program delivery, and the content of the curriculum. The two major targets for intervention have been the infant and the mother. The major program delivery forms have included home visitation, day care, parent group sessions, and job training. Curriculum content cannot be divided into distinct categories but has varied across a wide spectrum and includes content as diverse as sensorimotor infant exercises and parent problem solving skills.

Figure 1 provides a summary of program variations based on four forms of delivery. (For the sake of brevity, projects have been identified by the most convenient and familiar option: senior investigator, project location, or project name.) As seen from the figure, the largest number of programs were carried out through home visitation while day care was the second largest service delivery form. From Figure 1 seven different program types can be identified from the combinations of the four forms of delivery. Intervention programs that fall within each of these seven categories will be reviewed below. Since many of the references cited were published well after the projects were completed, the figure also provides the calendar years in which the researched intervention actually occurred for each project. Two

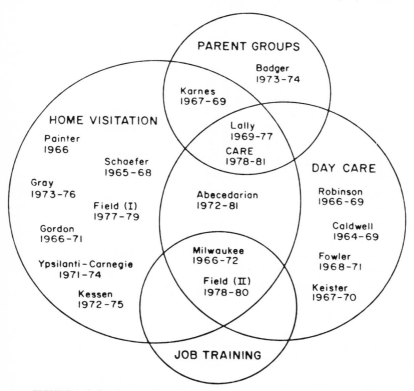

FIGURE 1. Infant intervention strategies and inclusive dates of implementation.

of the projects, CARE and Abecedarian, are still in operation in the research phase and plan to continue for several years. Others, such as Badger's and Keister's, have completed their research phase but continue as service projects.

Parent Group Sessions

Using a group meeting format for parents, Badger (1981) tested the feasibility of educational intervention within a large medical center. She recruited teen mothers who, along with their infants, attended weekly classes until the children were 18 months of age. The group training sessions helped mothers foster sensorimotor, cognitive and language development of their infants through an education curriculum (Badger, in press). Through group interaction the sessions provided a forum for discussion of many other family topics. The mothers and infants in these group training sessions were compared to a control group of mothers and infants who received monthly home visits that were supportive but did not include an infant curriculum component. Badger concluded that the cost of intervention favored a group approach.

Parent Group Sessions Plus Home Visitation

In an early study, Karnes and her associates in Illinois (Karnes, Teska, Hodgins, & Badger, 1970) provided a program of weekly two-hour parent meetings in an intervention lasting seven months. Unlike the Badger program, the children who were an average of 20 months of age at entry, did not come with their parents to the group sessions. The Karnes intervention was focused on helping the mother learn teaching techniques to use with the child and on topics of general interest such as discipline and birth control. Parents were provided with toys and educational materials to take home and were visited once a month to reinforce the group instruction. Thus, with the addition of minimal home visitation, the Karnes program can be viewed as a hybrid. Whereas home visits were used only once a month in her program, in other intervention programs home visits were used with much greater frequency, ranging from weekly to daily.

Home Visitation

Home visitation has been the delivery form most used by early interventionists. Two intense home visit programs conducted in the 1960s had the child as the primary target. Visitors in each of these programs went to the home for one hour a day, five days a week, and provided a structured program of stimulation for the child. The tutoring sessions of Schaefer and Aaronson (1977) in Washington, D.C. began when the infant reached 15 months of age and continued through 36 months of age. This time was chosen because it had previously been shown to be a period of first intellectual decline for disadvantaged children (Golden et al., 1971). Painter's (1969) program in Illinois consisted of children eight to 24 months old who received tutoring for a period of one year. This was an extension of Kirk's (1958) remedial program to the area of prevention with high-risk children. The curriculum content of the Painter program was organized around stimulation of the five senses (Painter, 1971), whereas the Schaefer/Aaronson content was organized around a variety of subject topics and child skills (Furfey, Note 2). The fact that no home visit programs implemented at a later time maintained an exclusive focus on the child was probably due to Schaefer's abandonment of this intervention strategy and his call for a broader approach to early education (Schaefer, 1970, 1972).

Gray's family-oriented home visiting program (Gray & Ruttle, 1980) began, like Schaefer and Aaronson's, when one child in the family was a toddler. Families containing two or three preschoolers were chosen because Gray's earlier research (Gray & Klaus, 1970) had suggested that intervention could have a family-wide and continuing effect. Unlike the programs of Schaefer and of Painter, this intervention focused on the mother, with child involvement allowed but not emphasized. The curriculum (Hardge & Gray, Note 3) was delivered in nine months of weekly visits planned to be specific to each family and its particular constellation of children.

Field's home-delivered intervention (Field, Widmayer, Stringer, & Ignatoff, 1981) began when the children were younger than Gray's and the shorter visits were spread out over a longer period of time. Biweekly visits beginning soon after birth and continuing for a year and a half were provided for teenage mothers. The delivery strategy further increased the focus on the mother by having the professional visitor accompanied by an aide whose job was to play with other children in the family in order to keep them from distracting the visit process. At each visit, the adolescent mother was taught sensorimotor, caretaking, and interaction exercises to use with her baby.

Three major home visitation programs contained internal variations so that, in effect, one program strategy was compared against the other. In the oldest of these interventions, Gordon (Olmsted, Rubin, True, & Revicki, Note 4) used weekly visits by a trained paraprofessional, but varied the age at which children entered the visitation program and the length of time they remained there. Some children entering at three months were involved in the program for as long as three years. The intervention was targeted for both the mother and the infant. The program objectives were to enhance intellectual and personality development of the child and to positively influence the mother's self-esteem. Curriculum content descriptions focused on Piagetian games (Gordon, 1970), preschool activities (Gordon, Guinagh, & Jester, 1972), and mother-infant interaction (Gordon, 1978). A unique feature of the Gordon program was that some children at age two were included in a Home Learning Center where they received social experiences in groups of five to supplement the individual visitation program.

The Ypsilanti-Carnegie infant program (Lambie, Bond, & Weikart, 1974) also varied the entry age of the children but over a much narrower range. Their weekly visits, lasting from 60 to 90 minutes, focused on the mother and had an overall objective to help mothers adopt a teaching style that supported their child's learning and growth. Whereas some projects produced curriculum guide books, this one documented its program with video tapes (High/Scope, Note 5).

Kessen and Fein (1975) varied their treatment in terms of curriculum content and intervention target rather than entry age or duration of intervention. All children were admitted at 12 months of age and the program lasted until they were 30 months old. For all children the visits began on a weekly basis and were then phased down to a bi-weekly and finally a monthly basis. Visitor, mother, and child were involved as a triad in each of three curriculum content variations (Fein, 1976), respectively emphasizing play, language, and social development. Some content from all three of these curricula was put together to form two other treatments that varied according to the intervention target. In the first of these, the visitor focused on the mother only and in the second focused on the child only. The fact that these complex variations of content and target produced only a modest and temporary variation in outcome reveals the limitations of our present methodologies in carrying out research on subtle differences in curriculum content. Methodologies have been more successfully adapted to the study of variables such as intensity (for example, dramatic differences in durations, as in Gordon's intervention) or breadth (for example, Gray's family-oriented program).

Home Visitation Plus Parent Groups and Group Day Care

Two programs created a broad intervention by combining individual home visits with parent group meetings and infant group day care. In the earlier of these (Lally & Honig, 1977), the home visits started during the last three months of the mother's pregnancy. During the visits, the trainers included demonstrations of learning games (Lally & Gordon, 1977) and modeling of positive teaching styles. The infants were six months of age before they were admitted to the day care center, and the home visitors continued to act as a liaison between the center and the parent, providing group meetings on topics of concern or interest to parents. Project CARE (Ramey, Sparling, & Wasik, 1981) used the same three-way combination but did not start the visits or group meetings until the infants entered day care at about three months of age. A second group in Project CARE received only two components of the intervention: parent group meetings and home visitation which contained a planned curriculum of infant learning games, parent problem solving skills and other parenting topics.

Home Visitation Plus Group Day Care

The timing for the home visitation element of the Abecedarian Project (Ramsey & Haskins, 1981) was almost the opposite of Lally's strategy. Home visitation was not used at all during the preschool years when group day care was provided. During these early years, the intervention program depended totally on an educational treatment embedded in a day care service (Sparling & Lewis, 1981a, 1981b; Ramey, McGinness, Cross, Collier, & Barrie-Blackley, in press). It was not until the end of the preschool period that a home visitation component was added for half of the subjects to act as a liaison between the public school and the parent. Whereas the Lally strategy emphasized the transition from home to center, the Abecedarian strategy focused on the transition from center to public school.

Home Visitation Plus Day Care and Job Training

The Milwaukee intervention (Garber & Heber, 1977), like Lally's program, began with home visitation. These were extended daily visits until the infant was four months of age when day care began. This intervention was aimed at preventing mental retardation in the offspring of high risk families. Thus the specific infant curriculum focus was on those areas (e.g., language, problem solving, and motivation) in which the mildly retarded and severely disadvantaged have often been found deficient (Garber, 1977). In addition to day care, a program of job training or vocational rehabilitation was provided for the mothers of the day care infants. The actual vocational and rehabilitation program was conducted only during the first years of the project, but parent support counseling continued. The intensity of the program should be credited as a major element of this intervention. Staff for visitation and day care began on a 1:1 child/adult ratio and never rose above 3:1. Regardless of form, target, or content, this makes the Milwaukee program the most intensive of those reviewed.

A more recent intervention of lesser intensity (Field, Widmayer, Greenberg, & Stollen, Note 6) also combined the elements of center day care and mother job training, but went one step further by comparing this combined treatment with a separate home visitation program for mothers and their infants. Those adolescent mothers receiving the home-based intervention were visited bi-weekly and provided training in infant stimulation: caretaking, sensorimotor, and interaction exercises. The mothers of the infants who received day care were involved in paid CETA job training as teacher aides in the same nursery that cared for their own children. While this program lasted only six months, it demonstrated a creative combination of intervention strategies which could keep mother and child together while providing differentiated help for each.

Group Day Care

Four interventions kept their delivery strategy almost solely within the boundaries of day care. The first two of these (Caldwell & Richmond, 1968; Keister, Note 7) exerted broad influence on the general practice of group day care for very young children. When these projects began in the 1960s, few early childhood professionals considered group day care for infants and toddlers to be benign, let along beneficial. These demonstrations did much to allay some of the fears based on unwarranted generalizations from the institutionalization literature to the day care field. Keister demonstrated that quality day care was not detrimental to infants and toddlers. This center disavowed any formal "curriculum" in its day care program, yet the program description (Keister, Note 7) showed that group care facilitated by well trained professionals could be made up of many rich experiences.

Caldwell's program contained a more structured plan and like others that followed (Fowler, 1972; Robinson & Robinson, 1971) showed that quality group day care could be not only without harm, but could positively benefit some children. The Robinsons put together a program in which children were cared for in multi-aged groups and received instructions from specialized teachers in topics such as language, pre-reading, art, and foreign language. Fowler's demonstration project in infant day care developed a curriculum organized around three forms of activity: (a) day care routines, (b) free play, and (c) guided learning in interactive play (Fowler, 1972). The degree of specification this program gave to the curriculum content and approach (Fowler, 1980a; 1980b) stands as an original contribution to the intervention literature.

Design and Results

This section will focus on the design and results of the early intervention programs. In Table 1 information on the design and outcome of all 18 studies covered in this article are presented. The studies themselves are grouped according to three major strategies of research design: single treatment with randomly assigned subjects to experimental or control groups; single treatment with matched control subjects; and multiple treatment comparisons with random assignment and controls. The following specific topics related to design and results will be covered: sample size, sample composition, attrition, repeated measures and significance testing, evaluation measures, replications, and continuing and delayed effects.

Sample Size

Sample size in these programs is usually small; programs are costly and recruitment of many subjects over a short period of time is often difficult. Small sample size is a concern in interpreting intervention results. As Stedman and his colleagues cautioned in 1972, ''Most projects have an insufficient sample size to base the extent of trust and credibility on their outcomes that is leading us to massive intervention service program'' (Stedman et al., Note 1, p. 8).

In order to obtain a larger sample size, recruitment of subjects can take place over a longer period of time and subjects can be brought in as separate cohorts. Any study following this procedure needs to report measures on cohorts to establish comparability of groups. Both the program by Gordon (1978) and the Abecedarian Project (Ramey, Holmberg, Sparling, & Collier, 1977) recruited over time and also reported comparison data on cohorts.

Sample Composition

The composition of the sample in most of the studies is heavily weighted towards the low socioeconomic segment of the population, and in many of the studies the majority of the subjects are black. This fact may limit the generalization of the findings.

There is a problem of self-selection with all of these programs involving disadvantaged families. Every project had a certain number of mothers who did not agree to participate when asked. Some who initially agreed to participate later declined because of the group to which they were assigned. Therefore, projects may have had mothers who were relatively more cooperative and motivated.

Table 1

Design and Results of Infant Invervention Studies

Director and Name of Project	Form of Program	Age at Entry	Number	Demographic Characteristics	Group Assignment	Results[a]
B. Caldwell, The Children's Center, Syracuse (early study)	Day care	7-43 months	78 in E; 61 in C	Wide range SES; black and white	Began recruiting C subjects about 1 year after Es	E>C on gain scores (+13 for E; -7 for C), but not on absolute scores (115 for E; 106 for C). No group differences in attachment to mother.
R. Lally and A. Honig, The Children's Center, Syracuse	Day care + HV	6 months	108 Es entered; 75 completed 4 years, only 38 through 6 years	Lower SES; black and white; family income < $5000; mother education <12th; unemployed to semiskilled	At 36 months recruited matched controls and some middle income Ss	E>C on SB at 36 and 40 months, but not at 60 or 72 months. Similar pattern on ITPA scores. E>C on several school behavior ratings. E>C on HOME scores at 48 months, but not 60 months.
G. Painter, Structured Tutorial Program	Home visits (HV)	8-24 months	30	Lower SES; black and white	Non-randomly assigned so as to distribute age, sex, and race between groups.	E>C on post-test SB. E>C on ITPA, many language tests and visual items, but only some reached significance.
W. Fowler, Ontario Institute for Studies of Education	Day care	2-30 months; mean = 7 months	39 Es 16 Cs	Broad range SES; black and white; only 9 were "culturally disadvantaged"	Recruited home-reared control Ss and matched in pairs on age, sex, parent education and Bayleys.	E>C on post-test IQ (SB or Bayley). Those who entered day care early (<14 months) had higher MDIs. Both E and C groups improved in language and socioemotional ratings.
M. Keister, Demonstration Project in Group Care of Infants	Day care	3 months	22	Middle and lower SES; black and white	Controls matched on age, sex, race, parent education, and birth order	No differences between E and C Ss on Bayley, Vineland or Preschool Attainment Record.
E. Badger, Infant Stimulation Mother Training Project	Parent groups in hospital vs. HV control	1 month	48; lost 6/12 white Ss; analysis on black Ss only	Lower SES; 36 black, 12 white; had to be on welfare and live ≤ 3 miles from hospital	12 Ss = 18 or 19 years. 12 Ss ≤ 16 years. Assigned to group meetings (E). Another 24 assigned to monthly HV control (C)	Among teenagers E>C on Bayley and Uzgiris-Hunt. No differences for children of older mothers. At 3 year follow-up, no McCarthy differences, but E>C on return to work/school and E<C on repeat pregnancies.

Table 1 (continued)

Director and Name of Project	Form of Program	Age at Entry	Number	Demographic Characteristics	Group Assignment	Results[a]
M. Karnes, J. Teska, A. Hodgins, and E. Badger, Mother's Training Program	Parent groups + HV	13-27 months	20 entered; 15 completed	Lower SES; black; family income <$4000; mean mother education =9.5 years	Control group recruited at end of study; matched by age, sex, race and other demographic factors	EXC on SR (16 points) and ITPA. Compared 6 Es to their older sibs who were tested before the study; Es were 28 points higher on the SB.
H. Robinson and N. Robinson, Frank Porter Graham Center	Day care	4 weeks-6 months	19	Broad range of SES; black and white	Recruited daycare group then later a group of 11 matched Controls.	At 18 months EXC on Bayley MDI; at 24 months EXC by 16 points on SB, but not significant because of low n.
E. Schaefer, Infant Education Research Project	HV	15 months	64 entered; 58 at 36 months; 48 at 1 year follow-up	Black; family income <$5000; mother education <12th; unskilled or semi-skilled	Randomly assigned to E or C group by neighborhood	At 36 months, EXC on SB, PPVT, and a perceptual test; at 1-year follow-up (48 months) E scores had dropped, so no significant group differences.
S. Gray, Family-oriented Home Visitor Program	HV	17-24 months	47 entered; 37 completed	Low SES; 1/2 black, 1/2 white; income <$4137; had to have sib <5 years old; mother non-working or worked at night	Randomly assigned to E or C group (Had a materials only group, but dropped analysis on them)	When toddlers, EXC on Bayley and Receptive Language Test. Mothers in EXC on cue labels and HOME. Two years later, differences sustained.
T. Field, Intervention for Prematurely Born Offspring of Teenage Mothers	HV	Birth	60 in E & C; 90 others in contrast groups	Low SES; black; teenage = mother <19 years; E and C babies were preterm	Randomly assigned to E or C	At 12 months EXC on Bayley MDIs and temperament ratings. Mothers talked to them more and E babies vocalized and played more. At 8 months EXC on HOME scores.
C. Ramey, J. Sparling, et al., Carolina Abecedarian Project	Day care + HVs at school age	6 weeks-3 months	116 entered; 104 still participating	Low SES; 98% black; high-risk score >11; mean income=$1455; mother education=10.2; IQ=84.2	Randomly assigned to E or C	EXC on Bayley, SB and WPPSI through 60 months. At 3 years EXC on language scores. In interactions, Es communicate to their mothers and modify more. No differences in mother attitudes or HOME scores.

Table 1 (continued)

Director and Name of Project	Form of Program	Age at Entry	Number	Demographic Characteristics	Group Assignment	Results[a]
R. Heber and H. Garber, Infant Education Center, Milwaukee Project	HV through 4 months then Day care + job training	Birth	40	Lower SES; black; IQ of 40 mothers <75	Assigned 1st 3 or 4 to E; next 3 or 4 to C.	E>C on all IQ tests after 12 months, and on ITPA and other language and problem solving tests. E mothers >C mothers in employment and self-confidence, and more responsive and verbal in interactions with child.
Gutelius, et al.	HV + Group Meetings + Medical Care	Birth	92	Lower SES; black; teen-age mother	Randomly assigned to E or C	E>C on S-B at 36 months, E mothers greater than C mothers in education and employment.
W. Kessen and G. Fein, Home-based Infant Education	HV (5 types)	12 months	108	90% white; most had high school education, few college; white and blue collar workers	Randomly assigned to 1 of 6 groups; Play, Language, or Social curriculum, Child-focus, Mother-focus, or Control	Language curriculum produced most improvement between 12-24 months, but by 30 months, no group differences. No change in maternal responsiveness which was correlated significantly with child competence. Families with extensive kin were more responsive to the program.
I. Gordon, Parent Education Program	HV until age 2; then Home Learning Center (HLC) +HV for some	3 months; Contrast group entered at 2 years	150 E; 60 C; Lost 13 by end of intervention and more at each follow-up	Urban and rural poor; 80% black	Randomly assigned to E or C in 1st year; then 1/2 assigned to C; from 24-36 months, 1/2 assigned to HLC or C	Program ended at age 3; at 6 years E>C on SB. At 2nd-4th grade follow-ups, E<C in special education placement; and E>C in reading, math, and problem solving. At age 10, Es in program 2 consecutive years or more > Cs on WISC-R.

Table 1 (continued)

T. Field, Mailman Center, Miami	HV vs. day care + job training vs. control	Birth	120 entered; 94 at 2 year follow-up	Lower SES; black; mothers <19 and had to enroll in CETA to be paid for day care work	Randomly assigned to 1 of 3 groups: Day care + training, HV or Controls	At 2 years Day care > HV>C on Bayley MDI, PDI and weight. Same pattern for mother's return to work/school and fewer repeat pregnancies. At 8 months, Day care Ss had more optimal temperament ratings. Never found HOME differences.
C. Ramey, J. Sparling and B. Wasik, Project CARE	Day care + HV vs. HV Alone vs. Control	6 weeks-3 months	82	63 low SES families; High-risk Index >11; 19 non-high-risk families; black and white	Randomly assigned to 1 of 3 groups: Day care + HV, HV, or Control	Project ongoing, oldest child not yet 4. 12 and 24 month Bayleys show Daycare > both other groups.
D. Lambie, J. Bond, and D. Weikart, Ypsilanti Carnegie Infant Education Project	2 types of HVs vs. Controls	3, 7, and 11 months	88 entered; 64 completed	Lower SES; mother's score on Ypsilanti SES scale <11	Randomly assigned to 1 of 3 groups: Professional HV, (E), Community visitors (CV) Controls (C)	At end of project, HV>CV on Bayley. At 1-year follow-up, no differences on SB. No HOME differences. E mothers >C on verbal interaction which correlated significantly with MDI. Age of entry made no difference.

Note. E=experimental; C=control; SB=Stanford-Binet; MDI=Mental Development Index; PDI=Psychomotor Development Index; HOME=Home Observation for Measurement of the Environment; ITPA=Illinois Test of Psycholinguistic Ability; PPVT=Peabody Picture Vocabulary Test; WPPSI=Wechsler Preschool and Primary Scale of Intelligence; WISC-R=Wechsler Intelligence Scale for Children-Revised

aAll differences reported (e.g. E>C) are statistically significant differences, unless otherwise noted.

73

Although subject samples may seem equally disadvantaged according to some risk index or income/occupation criterion, their levels of family functioning might be quite different. Thus, the cultural differences among disadvantaged groups may lead to different reactions to intervention. For example, Kessen and Fein (1975) reported that regardless of social class, families with extensive kin relations or expanded households were far more responsive to the intervention program than were families who had restricted social ties.

Comparison Groups

The majority of the studies include a test-only comparison group, whether randomly assigned or selected from another sample and matched with the subjects receiving treatment. Randomization is definitely preferred but, with small samples, randomization may not adequately assure initial equivalence of groups.

Several studies included multiple treatment groups, all of which used random subject assignment. For example, Kessen and Fein (1975) conducted a six-group comparison with 18 subjects in each group receiving the same treatment for 18 months. Gordon also had a multiple treatment program in which subjects received a home visit intervention for their first or second year of life or both years. Half of them later received a Home Learning Center plus Home Visit intervention for the third year. Including the initial controls and a contrast group recruited at age two, there were seven groups in all (Gordon, 1978). These multiple group studies require larger numbers of subjects, low attrition rates, and more complex data analyses.

Attrition

Subject attrition is typically a problem in these intervention studies. Consequently, tests of the equivalence of initial and final samples is particularly important to investigate the possibility that the resulting sample may not be representative of the initial sample (Schaie, 1965). Lally and Honig (1977), for example, used a trend analysis to show similar attrition patterns in the control and experimental groups. Even with such techniques, the composition of the group remaining in the study may be different on some crucial, yet unmeasured, characteristics.

Repeated Measures and Significance Testing

The repeated measures design of these projects requires special consideration in data management and analysis. For example, continuous assessment of control groups may in itself lead to some increases in scores, although

Haskins, Ramey, Stedman, Blacher-Dixon, and Pierce (1978) reported that this is not a crucial concern during infancy. Also, because of the number of analyses performed in longitudinal studies, the traditional .05 level of significance may be reached by chance a certain number of times. As a result Gray and Wandersman (1980) have suggested that more conservative alpha levels be used or data reduction techniques be employed to decrease the number of tests of significance for group differences.

Evaluation Measures

The outcome measures used in most studies are IQ scores. Yet standardized tests of intelligence may not be the best way to estimate the abilities of disadvantaged children. Such tests evaluate only a limited part of a child's functioning, albeit an important one.

Several attempts have been made to broaden the scope of evaluation measures. One example has been the assessment of parent-child interaction patterns as a function of early intervention. The most often used measure to investigate such changes is the Home Observation for Measurement of the Environment (HOME) (Bradley & Caldwell, 1976). It is a 45-question rating scale measuring interactions in the home and the quality of stimulation available to the child. Lally and Honig (1977), Gray and Ruttle (1980), Field et al. (1980), and Gordon and Guinagh (1978) have all reported increased home stimulation scores for their intervention groups, but not at all assessment periods.

Replications

Although some of these studies produced curricula that are widely used, few of them have been replicated in a standardized way. The Lally and Honig (1977) program was used in Kentucky in an 18-county project involving 3600 children. The basic concepts of the Syracuse intervention were exported to the Kentucky projects, but tight replications were not carried out (Stedman et al., Note 1). Badger (Note 8) identifies at least a dozen replications of her parent group meeting format, but data on these have not been published. It is appropriate to note that one related study does provide standardized procedures for replications, Levenstein's Verbal Interaction Project (Madden, Levenstein, & Levenstein, 1976). However, the children began participation in the project after infancy, and thus it is not included in this review.

Continuing and Delayed Effects

Intervention programs are criticized because their impact on children's performances seems to fade over time. Thus, it is important to assure that evaluation occurs over time and that follow-up measures are taken. The intervention phase has ended for all but two of the studies described in this review. (Both the Abecedarian Project and Project CARE in North Carolina are ongoing.) The follow-up evaluation phase for some of the projects does continue in order to measure potential long-term effects of intervention. A recent major follow-up of fourteen early intervention programs, not all of which dealt with infancy, has been reported by Darlington et al. (1980).

Three critical outcome areas are of particular interest in follow-up efforts: cognitive outcome of the child, parent or family effects, and later school performance of the child. Two interventions (Gray & Wandersman, 1980; Gordon & Guinagh, 1978) which focused on the parent/infant dyad through home visits have reported sustained child effects: the Gray project through age 4 and the Gordon project through age 10. As a measure of sustained effects on the family, Gray reported superior experimental group scores on Caldwell's HOME scale when children were 4 years old, two years after intervention. When the Gordon children were 6 years old, three years after intervention, he reported superior experimental group scores on the Home Environment Rating (HER), a scale developed in the Gordon project. Furthermore, HER scores at age six predicted child assignment to special education at age ten. Experimental subjects in the Gordon study had fewer special education placements in school and performed better on school achievement tests.

Three projects (Field, Note 6; Ramey & Haskins, 1980; Garber, 1979), each of which enhanced the intensity of treatment by combining at least two forms of intervention delivery, have shown continuing positive intellectual effects for children ages two, five, and ten respectively. (Project CARE also has a combined treatment group but it is only of two years' duration so long-term or follow-up results have not been reported.) Family effects were reported, by both Ramey and Garber, in the greater frequency with which mothers in the experimental groups returned to work or school and, by Field, in a lower rate of repeat pregnancies. Two of these studies have included job training for the mother, which suggests that changing the mother's situation in life, in combination with other supportive services, may contribute to the child's development.

Referring to the implementation dates in Figure 1, one can see that ten new programs began between 1964 and 1970. The rate of new program developments slowed in the next decade with only eight being initiated. The disillusionment with earlier findings most likely contributed to this decline in interest. However, later long-term follow-up data, especially those showing continuing or delayed effects (Darlington et al., 1980; Field, Note 6; Ramey & Haskins, 1980; Garber, 1979) suggest that renewed attention should be given to this field.

Since the completion of some of the earlier of these projects, several new theoretical positions have been articulated that have implications for infant intervention programs. For example, these new perspectives should help redefine critical variables for the prevention of cognitive and social handicapping conditions. In the next section, three significant theoretical developments will be examined.

Theoretical Perspectives with Implications for Infant Intervention

Based upon the pioneering work of these early projects, the field is now ready for the exploration of innovative variations on program design and evaluation. There are, however, some major new theoretical emphases or perspectives that should be taken into account as new programs are developed because each perspective has important implications for both infant program planning and evaluation. These three perspectives are (1) Bell's description of the bidirectional influence in mother-child relationship, (2) Sameroff and Chandler's transactional process, and (3) General Systems Theory as described by von Bertalanffy and by Miller.

The first of these perspectives is the one popularized by Bell (1974) and concerns the bidirectional influences in mother-infant relationships. The prevailing paradigm for studying dyadic interchanges has historically been a unidirectional model in which variations in caregiver interactional styles and attitudes have been assumed as causal agents in the individual differences in social and cognitive attributes of developing infants. Bell (1974) has pointed out that this simplistic notion of cause and effect has not done justice to the presenting or demand characteristics of infants which, in all probability, also influence the types of behaviors and attitudes that parents display toward their infants. In essence, Bell's argument reinforces Piaget's notion of the infant as an active organism and postulates that these differential demand characteristics are one way in which the infant contributes to the creation of his or her own caregiving environment. Thus, for example, infants with different temperamental characteristics may elicit different caregiving styles as well as be influenced unidirectionally by those different styles.

The second perspective is that of transactional processes as popularized by Sameroff and Chandler (1975). The idea of transactional processes implies that infants with different biological or psychological risk characteristics might have different developmental outcomes depending on the environments to which those risk characteristics are exposed. Thus, there is no necessary relationship between a predisposing condition, such as phenylketurnia or prematurity, and developmental outcome that is independent of the quality of the rearing and caregiving environment to which the infant is exposed.

Zeskind and Ramey (1978, 1981) have shown, for example, that fetal malnourishment is associated with developmental delay in infancy for lower-class infants who do not participate in an early intervention program, but similar infants are indistinguishable from well-nourished lower-class infants if they have received early educational intervention. An important observation was the fact that mothers of the fetally malnourished lower-class infants in the control group reduced their level of involvement with their infants, but this apparent consequence of fetal malnourishment was not observed in the mothers of children given early educational intervention. Thus, the Zeskind and Ramey studies provide experimental evidence both for Sameroff and Chandler's transactional process idea and for Bell's (1974) bidirectional influence notion.

The third major new construct comes from systems theory as described by von Bertalanffy (1975) and Miller (1978) in their General Systems Theory. A major concept within systems theory is the need to analyze how change in one part of the system effects change in another part.

Drawing upon the concepts of the levels of analysis principle and the concept of feedback embedded in General Systems Theory, Ramey, MacPhee, and Yeates (in press) have demonstrated that early intervention in the form of educational daycare affects not only the developmental level of the children but also has positive effects on mothers' educational attainment and employment compared to children and mothers in a randomly constituted control group. Thus, an intervention strategy focused primarily on infants and young children has had an indirect influence on the educational and occupational status of the child's mother. This finding illustrates that an intervention at one level of the family may affect not only the targeted level (in this case, the child), but may have reverberating and potentially lasting influences at other levels of family functioning.

Recommendations

Using the three theoretical perspectives described above and the conclusions of past and current programs, one can made recommendations for future planning and evaluation of prevention-oriented programs designed for high-risk infants. One can now ask what are the important knowledge gaps as a result of prior research and can direct future work towards gaining knowledge in these areas. Even though we have a large knowledge base compared to a few years ago, our understanding of the full consequences of early preventive efforts is inconclusive. One does not know the exact mechanisms through which these programs achieved their effects. Limited knowledge exists on side effects. Extremely little information exists on the relative benefits and costs of alternative preventive programs. Consequently, the three recommendations that follow contain strategies for gaining knowledge in these areas.

First, assessment should be process oriented as well as product oriented. Early intervention programs should focus on an assessment over time of the psychological and biological mechanisms targeted for change rather than focusing exclusively on measuring outcome or output variables. Thus, for example, if a home-based prevention oriented program has targeted early mother-infant social interactions as the primary mechanism for changing the infant's development, then changes in those variables should be as much the focus of the evaluation plan as the developmental status of the child.

Information about processes will allow a more precise determination of why some programs are successful in meeting their objectives whereas others are not. Such an orientation will also highlight the basic research contributions possible through applied research by bringing under experimental consideration the mechanisms thought to be causally implicated in the development of young children and their families. Such an orientation will typically require a time series or repeated measures analysis. Such analyses are not often used as a research strategy in the study of child and family development generally, yet they have been repeatedly demonstrated to be a powerful experimental design.

Second, a multi-level evaluation strategy is recommended. Such a strategy involves measuring several variables simultaneously. To the extent that families of high-risk children are nested in a complex web of ecologies, as Bronfenbrenner (1975) suggests, then attempting to alter one or more components of a multilevel system, with feedback across levels, should sensitize us to potential ripple effects from our interventions. Given that unintended side effects may be both positive and negative, it is all the more apparent that comprehensive evaluations are practically and ethically essential.

Finally, it is recommended that technically adequate experimental comparisons of alternative forms of prevention-oriented services for high-risk infants be conducted. The five direct comparison studies included in this review reveal the tentativeness with which this task has been thus far undertaken. In the absence of direct, experimental comparisons, cost-benefit analyses of alternative forms of early intervention are difficult, if not impossible. In an age of increased economic pressures on the delivery of human services, the country can ill-afford not to have this important information which is an essential ingredient for rational and humane social service policy.

REFERENCE NOTES

1. Stedman, D. J., Anastasiow, N. J., Dokecki, P. R., Gordon, I. J., & Parker, R. K. *How can effective early intervention programs be delivered to potentially retarded children?* A report for the Office of the Secretary of the Department of Health, Education and Welfare, October, 1972.

2. Furfey, P. H. (Ed.). *Education of children aged one to three: A curriculum manual* (Infant Education Research Project). Unpublished manuscript, The Catholic University of America, 1972.

3. Hardge, B., & Gray, S. *Helping families learn: A home-based program* (Demonstration and Research Center for Early Education). Unpublished manuscript, Peabody College, Vanderbilt University, 1975.

4. Olmsted, P. O., Rubin, R. I., True, J. H., Revicki, D. A. *Parent education: The contributions of Ira J. Gordon.* Booklet, 1980. (Available from the Association for Childhood Education International, 3615 Wisconsin Ave. N.W., Washington, D. C. 20016).

5. High/Scope Educational Research Foundation. *Audio-visual materials.* Catalog. (Available from High/Scope Educational Research Foundation, 600 North River St., Ypsilanti, MI 48197).

6. Field, T., Widmayer, S., Greenberg, R., & Stollen, S. *Effects of parent training on teenage mothers and their infants.* Final report to the Administration for Children, Youth, and Families, 1981.

7. Keister, M. E. *"The good life" for infants and toddlers.* Booklet, 1970. (Available from National Association for the Education of Young Children, 1834 Connecticut Ave. N.W., Washington, D. C. 20009).

8. Badger, E. Personal communication, May 19, 1981.

REFERENCES

Badger, E. *Infant-toddler: Introducing your child to the joy of learning.* New York: McGraw-Hill, in press.

Badger, E. Effects of parent education program on teenage mothers and their offspring. In K. G. Scott, T. Field, & E. Robertson (Eds.), *Teenage parents and their offspring.* New York: Grune & Stratton, 1981.

Bell, R. Q. Contributions of human infants to caregiving and social interaction. In M. Lewis & R. A. Rosenblum (Eds.), *The effect of the infant on its caregiver.* New York: John Wiley & Sons, 1974.

Bertalanffy, L. V. *Perspectives on general system theory.* New York: George Braziller, 1975.

Bradley, R., & Caldwell, B. Early home environment and changes in mental test performance in children 6 to 36 months. *Developmental Psychology*, 1976, *12*, 93–97.

Bronfenbrenner, U. Is early intervention effective? In M. Guttentag & E. L. Struening (Eds.), *Handbook of evaluation research* (Vol. 2), Beverly Hills: Sage Publications, 1975.

Caldwell, B. M., & Richmond, J. B. The Children's Center in Syracuse, New York. In L. L. Dittman (Ed.), *Early child care: The new perspectives.* New York: Atherton Press, 1968.

Darlington, R. B., Royce, J. M., Snipper, A. S., Murray, H. W., & Lazar, I. Preschool programs and later school competence of children from low-income families. *Science*, 1980, *208*, 202–204.

Fein, G. (Ed.) Social organization and the development of the individual. In K. F. Riegal & J. A. Meacheam (Eds.), *The developing individual in a changing world.* The Hague: Mouton, 1976.

Field, T. Early development of the preterm offspring of teenage mothers. In K. G. Scott, T. Field, & E. Robertson (Eds.), *Teenage parents and their offspring.* New York: Grune & Stratton, 1981.

Field, T., Widmayer, S., Stringer, S., & Ignatoff, E. Teenage, lower-class black mothers and their preterm infants: An intervention and developmental follow-up. *Child Development*, 1980, *51*, 426–436.

Fowler, W. A developmental learning approach to infant care in a group setting. *Merrill-Palmer Quarterly*, 1972, *18*, 145–175.

Fowler, W. *Curriculum and assessment guides for infant and child care*. Boston: Allyn & Bacon, 1980. (a)

Fowler, W. *Infant and child care: A guide to education in group settings*. Boston: Allyn & Bacon, 1980. (b)

Garber, H. L. Preventing mental retardation through family rehabilitation. In B. M. Caldwell & D. J. Stedman (Eds.), *Infant education: A guide for helping handicapped children in the first three years*. New York: Walker & Co., 1977.

Garber, H. L. Bridging the gap from preschool to school for the disadvantaged child. *School Psychology Digest*, 1979, *8*, 303–310.

Garber, H., & Heber, R. The Milwaukee Project: Indications of the effectiveness of early intervention in preventing mental retardation. In P. Mittler (Ed.), *Research to practice in mental retardation: Care and intervention* (Vol. 1). Baltimore: University Park Press, 1977.

Golden, M., Birns, B., Bridger, W., & Moss, A. Social-class differentiation in cognitive development among black preschool children. *Child Development*, 1971, *42*, 37–45.

Gordon, I. *Baby learning through baby play: A parent guide for the first two years*. New York: St. Martin's Press, 1970.

Gordon, I. *Baby to parent, parent to baby: A guide to loving and learning in a child's first year*. New York: St. Martin's Press, 1978.

Gordon, I. J., Guinagh, B., & Jester, R. E. *Child learning through child play*. New York: St. Martin's Press, 1972.

Gordon, I. J., & Guinagh, B. J. A home learning center approach to early stimulation. *JSAS Catalog of Selected Documents in Psychology*, 1978, *8*, 6. (Ms. No. 1634).

Gray, S. W., & Klaus, R. A. The early training project: A seventh year report. *Child Development*, 1970, *41*, 909–924.

Gray, S. W., & Ruttle, K. The family-oriented home visiting program: A longitudinal study. *Genetic Psychology Monographs*, 1980, *102*, 299–316.

Gray, S. W., & Wandersman, L. P. The methodology of home-based intervention studies: Problems and strategies. *Child Development*, 1980, *51*, 993–1009.

Haskins, R., Finkelstein, N. W., & Stedman, D. J. Infant-stimulation programs and their effects. *Pediatric Annals*, 1978, *7*, 99–128.

Haskins, R., Ramey, C. T., & Stedman, D. J., Blacher-Dixon, J., & Pierce, J. E. Effects of repeated assessment on standardized test performance by infants. *American Journal of Mental Deficiency*, 1978, *83* (3), 233–239.

Hunt, J. McV. *Intelligence and experience*. New York: Ronald Press Company, 1961.

Itard, J. M. G. [*The wild boy of Aveyron*] (G. & M. Humphrey, trans.), New York: Appleton-Century-Crofts, 1932. (Originally published, 1894.)

Karnes, M. B., Teska, J. A., Hodgins, A. S., & Badger, E. D. Educational intervention at home by mothers of disadvantaged infants. *Child Development*, 1970, *41*, 925–935.

Kessen, W., & Fein, G. *Variations in home-based infant education: Language, play and social development. Final Report*. New Haven, Conn.: Yale University Press, 1975. (ERIC Document Reproduction Service No. ED 118 233)

Kirk, S. A. *Early education of the mentally retarded: An experimental study*. Urbana, Illinois: University of Illinois Press, 1958.

Kirk, S. A., & Gallagher, J. J. *Educating exceptional children* (3rd ed.). Boston, Mass.: Houghton Mifflin Company, 1979.

Lally, J. R., & Gordon, I. J. *Learning games for infants and toddlers*. Syracuse, New York: New Readers Press, 1977.

Lally, J. R., & Honig, A. S. The family development research program. In M. C. Day & R. Parker (Eds.), *The preschool in action*. New York: Allyn & Bacon, 1977.

Lambie, D. Z., Bond, J. T., & Weikart, D. P. *Home teaching with mothers and infants: The Ypsilanti-Carnegie Infant Education Project—An experiment.* Ypsilanti, Michigan: High/Scope Educational Research Foundation, 1974.

Madden, J., Levenstein, P., & Levenstein, S. Longitudinal IQ outcomes of the mother-child home program. *Child Development*, 1976, *46*, 1015–1025.

Mercer, J. R. *System of multicultural pluralistic assessment, technical manual.* New York: The Psychological Corporation, 1979.

Miller, J. G. *Living systems.* New York: McGraw-Hill, 1978.

Painter, G. The effect of a structured tutorial program on the cognitive and language development of culturally disadvantaged infants. *Merrill-Palmer Quarterly*, 1969, *15*, 279–294.

Painter, G. *Teach your baby.* New York: Simon and Schuster, 1971.

Ramey, C. T., & Campbell, F. A. Compensatory education for disadvantaged children. *School Review*, 1979, *87*, 171–189.

Ramey, C. T., & Haskins, R. The causes and treatment of school failure: Insights from the Carolina Abecedarian Project. In M. Begab, H. Garber, & H. C. Haywood (Eds.), *Causes and prevention of retarded development in psychosocially disadvantaged children.* Baltimore: University Park Press, 1981.

Ramey, C. T., Holmberg, M. C., Sparling, J. J., & Collier, A. M. An introduction to the Carolina Abecedarian Project. In B. M. Caldwell & D. J. Stedman (Eds.), *Infant education: A Guide for helping handicapped children in the first three years.* New York: Walker & Co., 1977, 101–121.

Ramey, C. T., MacPhee, D., & Yeates, K. O. Preventing developmental retardation: A general systems model. In L. Bond & J. Joffee (Eds.), *Facilitating infant and early childhood development.* Hanover, N. H.: University Press of New England, in press.

Ramey, C. T., McGinness, G. D., Cross, L., Collier, A., & Barrie-Blackley, S. The Abecedarian approach to social competence: Cognitive and linguistic intervention for disadvantaged preschoolers. In K. Borman (Ed.), *Socialization of the child in a changing society.* New York: Pergammon Press, in press.

Ramey, C. T., Sparling, J., & Wasik, B. H. Creating social environments to facilitate language development. In R. Scheifelbush & D. Bricker (Eds.), *Early language intervention.* Baltimore: University Park Press, 1981.

Robinson, H. B., & Robinson, N. M. Longitudinal development of very young children in a comprehensive day care program: The first two years. *Child Development*, 1971, *42*, 1673–1683.

Sameroff, A. J., & Chandler, M. J. Reproductive risk and the continuum of caretaking casualty. In F. D. Horowitz (Ed.), *Review of child development research* (Vol. 4). Chicago: University of Chicago Press, 1975.

Schaefer, E. S. Need for early and continuing education. In V. M. Dennenberg (Ed.), *Education of the infant and young child.* New York: Academic Press, 1970.

Schaefer, E. S. Parents as educators: Evidence from cross-sectional, longitudinal research. *Young Children*, 1972, *27*, 227–239.

Schaefer, E. S., & Aaronson, M. Infant Education Research Project: Implementation and implications of the home tutoring program. In M. E. Day & R. K. Parker (Eds.), *The preschool in action* (2nd ed.). Boston: Allyn and Bacon, 1977.

Schaie, L. W. A general model for the study of developmental problems. *Psychological Bulletin*, 1965, *64*, 92–107.

Skeels, H. M., & Dye, H. B. A study of the effects of differential stimulation on mentally retarded children. *Proceedings of the American Association on Mental Deficiency*, 1939, *44*, 114–136.

Sparling, J., & Lewis, I. *Learningames for the first three years: A guide to parent-child play.* New York: Berkley Books, 1981. (a)

Sparling, J., & Lewis, I. *Learningames for the first three years: A program for a parent/center partnership.* New York: Walker and Company, 1981. (b)

Westinghouse Learning Corporation. *The impact of Head Start: An evaluation of Head Start on children's cognitive and affective development.* Athens: Ohio University, 1969.

Zeskind, P., & Ramey, C. T. Fetal malnutrition: An experimental study of its consequences on infant development in two care-giving environments. *Child Development*, 1978, *49*, 115–1162.

Zeskind, P. S., & Ramey, C. T. Preventing intellectual and interactional sequelae of fetal malnutrition: A longitudinal, transactional and synergistic approach to development. *Child Development*, 1981.

A STRUCTURAL EQUATION MODEL ANALYSIS OF COMPETENCE IN CHILDREN AT RISK FOR MENTAL DISORDER

Ronald Seifer
Arnold J. Sameroff

ABSTRACT. Factors influencing the stability of child competence from 30 months to 48 months of age are investigated using structural equation model techniques in a population at presumed risk for mental disorder because their mothers have a diagnosed psychiatric disturbance. This method allows for the simultaneous analysis of many variables in testing hypotheses about causality in longitudinal investigations. Child competence was defined in terms of cognitive and social variables. Background environmental variables included were social class, race, and maternal psychopathology. Three models were examined in this study. The first model posited direct effects of child factors as well as effects of background environmental factors in the stability of child competence. The second model posited only effects of background variables, with no direct child effects. The third model posited child effects and a subset of the background effects in the first model. The second model, one that did not include direct child effects, was found to be the most parsimonious explanation of the data. This finding supports the position that interventions for children at risk be aimed at the social milieu in which individual children are embedded.

One of the fundamental issues in the development of preventive programs, an issue that is often not explicitly considered, is determining what should be the target of such interventions. In the case where preventive measures are directed to insuring that children with identified or potential developmental problems suffer the least possible insult, an obvious choice is most often made — to target intervention programs at the children in question. There is, however, an increasing realization that interventions aimed solely at children are less successful than one might hope. There are theoretical and empirical reasons to expect that such would be the case.

In their analysis of man-environment transactions, Wapner, Kaplan, and Cohen (1973) argue that one must understand complete systems of human

Reprints may be obtained from the authors at the Institute for the Study of Developmental Disabilities, University of Illinois at Chicago Circle, 1640 West Roosevelt Road, Chicago, IL 60608.

action in order to fully comprehend the way that individuals structure and develop in varied environments. They argue that individuals cannot be understood without reference to the actions they engage in, the instrumentalities available to them, the purposes of their activity, and the scene in which the activity occurs. Sameroff (1981) has also emphasized the need for an understanding of complete social systems for an adequate explanation of development. There is a need to transcend a rigid analysis of the individual and consider larger social systems that play a major role in the determination of individual behavior. The clear implication of such theoretical positions is that attempts to enhance the development of individual children cannot focus exclusively on those individuals without concurrent efforts to optimize the larger social scene.

On a more empirical note, Sameroff and Chandler (1975) documented the degree to which children who entered the world in a state of reproductive risk exhibited differential developmental outcomes as a function of their social context. It is not sufficient to simply categorize children as at-risk due to presumed constitutional deficits resulting from perinatal insult. Rather, developmental transactions between these infants and their caregiving environments provide a superior explanation for their eventual developmental status.

Although there is theoretical justification, and empirical evidence regarding long-term outcome, supporting the idea that interventions be targeted at social systems, there is precious little basic research evidence demonstrating the relations between infants at risk and their caregiving environments. In this paper we will present an approach that has directly shown the importance of the larger social context in explaining continuity in child behavior in a population of children at risk for mental disorder. Through the use of structural equation models, which simultaneously evaluate a complete theoretical structuring of a data set, we will show that the effects of background social variables are necessary in the explanation of continuity of child competence.

Structural Equation Models

Although the collection of longitudinal data allows for the examination of hypotheses which could not otherwise be evaluated, there are many technical problems encountered when attempting to analyze such data. One of the basic problems is pragmatic; the simultaneous analysis of even a few variables over time is complex. Standard regression models often cannot accommodate the complexity needed for such analysis. A second problem is more conceptual; longitudinal data is generally collected in order to analyze causal effects of variables at earlier time periods on variables at subsequent points in time. Most statistical techniques do not assume particular directions of effects among variables.

Until recently, the proposed solutions to such problems, most often path analysis and cross-panel correlation analysis, provided techniques which were not applicable to many real-life developmental research questions. These methods had undesirable statistical properties, and were of questionable conceptual value (Ragosa, 1979). However, further developments in structural equation models have solved many of the problems associated with previous methods (Joreskog & Sorbum, 1978; Joreskog, 1979; Ragosa, 1979). The basic idea of structural equation modelling is to test a set of causal hypotheses against a set of observed data, generally a correlation or covariance matrix. Thus, the technique does not conclusively test causal models, rather, it evaluates the relative merit of several hypotheses for explaining a set of data.

The structural equation model used, LISREL, was developed by Joreskog and Sorbum (Joreskog, 1973; Joreskog & Sorbum, 1978). The definition of a hypothesis to be tested entails two steps. First is to define a set of latent variables derived from the variables actually measured. This is analagous to the creation of factor scores from a set of measured test items. The second step is to define the causal relationships among the latent variables which are created by the model. The LISREL model also allows for the specification of relations among the measured variables to account for covariance among the measures. The strength of such a structural equation model is that it analyzes all of this information simultaneously and provides a single significance test of the adequacy of the defined hypothesis for describing the structure of the observed data.

Rochester Longitudinal Study

The Rochester Longitudinal Study (RLS) is an examination of children at risk for mental illness who were followed from birth through four years of age (Sameroff & Zax, 1978; Sameroff & Seifer, 1981). The children were considered at risk for mental illness because their mothers were suffering from mild to severe psychiatric disorders. There is an extensive literature documenting that children of schizophrenic mothers, who were the major focus of the RLS, are at 10 to 15 times greater risk for developing schizophrenia than children in the general population. In addition, they are at risk for a wide variety of other disorders so that about 50% of these children are expected to exhibit some form of illness during their life (Hanson, Gottesman, & Meehl, 1977). In addition to children of schizophrenic women, the RLS sample includes mothers with a variety of psychiatric diagnoses as well as a group of mothers with no mental illness.

The major social context variables considered in this paper, besides maternal psychopathology, are race and socioeconomic status. These two social status factors have been implicated in the development of many aspects of early cognitive and social competence (Golden & Birns, 1976; Lewis & Wilson, 1972). Social status is of particular interest in the examination of the transmission of mental disorders and schizophrenia in particular. Schizophrenia is a disorder found disproportionately in lower class populations, a situation that cannot be explained by simple constitutional variables (Kohn, 1973). Kohn (1969, 1973) has hypothesized that social status variables determine the degree to which vulnerable individuals will be able to withstand the stresses of everyday life. Lower class culture, according to Kohn, fosters the development of rigid cognitive values which restrict the individual's ability to deal with stressful life events. Thus, it is an aspect of high-order social systems, transmitted through individuals, which accounts for the increased incidence of schizophrenia in lower class populations.

In the RLS, mothers and children were examined on several occasions. The mothers were interviewed prior to the birth of their child regarding their mental health status and attitudes toward pregnancy. During the newborn period, obstetric data was collected and the infant was evaluated in the laboratory. At 4 and 12 months, the infant was evaluated in the laboratory, and mother-infant interaction was observed in the home. At 30 and 48 months, both mother and child participated in extensive laboratory assessments.

The fact that the RLS is a longitudinal study allows us to employ some relatively new techniques in the analysis of the data. A brief description of the technique used was presented above. The two basic questions investigated in this paper are: (1) Where does the cause for continuity in child competence lie, in the child or in the caregiving environment? and (2) What are the most salient characteristics of the family, its social status and racial background or the mental health of the mother?

Models Tested in the Rochester Longitudinal Study

Although numerous measures were obtained in the RLS, a small subset was selected for these preliminary structural analyses. In this way some clear hypotheses could be proposed and tested about the relation of behavior at two points in time. These variables included measures of child competence and the influence of three background variables describing maternal status.

Two broad measures were used to define child competence. The first of these was intelligence test performance. At 30 months of age, the children were administered the Bayley Scales of Infant Development. At 48 months, they were tested with the verbal scales of the Wechsler Preschool and Primary Scale of Intelligence (WPPSI). The second measure of child competence was the global rating from the Rochester Adaptive Behavior Inventory or RABI (Seifer, Sameroff, & Jones, 1981) administered at 30 and 48 months. The RABI is a ninety minute interview of mothers regarding their children's adaptive behavior in a variety of settings. At the conclusion of the interview, a global rating is assigned to the child on a five point scale which ranges from above average adaptation to seriously disturbed.

Three aspects of mothers' status are used as background variables. The first of these is SES, computed using a modification of Hollingshead's (1957) two factor system. Where only the father's education and occupation are included in Hollingshead's original scoring system, we averaged in the mother's educational background prior to computation of the final SES score. This was done to take into account the frequent discrepancies between the education of the two parents found in our sample. The second background variable is race, restricted to black or white. A small number of Puerto Rican families in our sample are not used in these analyses. The final background variable is the severity of the mother's illness. This was scored at the completion of an extensive psychiatric interview on a four point scale that ranged from no illness to severe and debilitating disorder.

The creation of a structural model involves specification of a set of latent variables and the relationships among them. The idea of latent variables is from classical test theory where it is assumed that psychological tests imperfectly measure underlying traits. Thus, one attempts to measure such traits in more than one way in order to eliminate various sources of measurement error. The resulting composite variables, analogous to factor scores, are the latent variables used in LISREL models (Joreskog & Sorbum, 1978). In schematic representations arrows from the latent to the measured variables indicate this relationship. Also, single-headed arrows between latent variables indicate causal relationships among them. Finally, it is necessary to specify covariance relationships among the measured variables which are independent of the latent variables. These are indicated by double-headed arrows which do not imply a direction of cause.

Such hypothesized causal models are tested by comparing the original correlation matrix of measured variables with a corresponding matrix created by the LISREL model. The latter matrix takes into account the causal links among the measured and latent variables hypothesized in the model. A chi-square statistic is obtained which indexes the amount of discrepancy between the original and derived matrices. Large, and significant, chi-square statistics indicate a large discrepancy, and thus a poor fit of the hypothesized model to the original data. In such cases the model is considered a poor description of the data. If the chi-square statistic is small, a non-significant discrepancy, the model is assumed to fit the data. Each individual path may be tested for significance using a t-statistic. If the model is a poor fit to the data, two steps are taken. First, discrepancies between the original data and the LISREL model are examined. Those relationships that show the most discrepancy are changed, i.e., added or subtracted, in the model. Second, those paths that do not show significant t-statistics are eliminated from the model. Both of these steps generally enhance the fit of the model to the original data.

The first model tested hypothesizes that all of the measures discussed above are important in the continuity of child competence. This model is presented graphically in Figure 1 and is referred to as Model 1. At both 30 and 48 months a latent variable is created from the intelligence test score and the RABI global rating. This is indicated by the arrows from "child competence" to the two measures at each age. The model also allows for intercorrelation between the RABI at 30 and 48 months and between intelligence test scores at 30 and 48 months, indicated by the double-headed arrows between these measures.

A third latent variable, mother status, is created from the SES, race, and severity of illness measures. These measures were stable over the 18 month time period, so that only one latent variable was necessary. It was also determined that the optimal hypothesis allowed for covariation between severity of illness and race, indicated by the arrow between them.

Once the latent variables are defined, causal paths among them are hypothesized in Model 1. First, the path from child competence at 30 months to child competence at 48 months indicates a direct influence of child variables from the first measurement period to the second. The two paths from mother status to child competence at each age indicate a direct influence of the background measures upon child competence.

Model 1 was tested and found to be unsatisfactory. The matrix of relationships among the variables produced by the model was found to differ substantially from the observed correlations among the measures. This resulted in a large and significant chi-square statistic (chi-square $=16.45$, df $= 8$, $p < .05$).

Examination of the discrepancy between the LISREL model and the original data matrix indicates two problems. First, the relationships between severity of illness and other measures under the hypothesis of Model 1 are

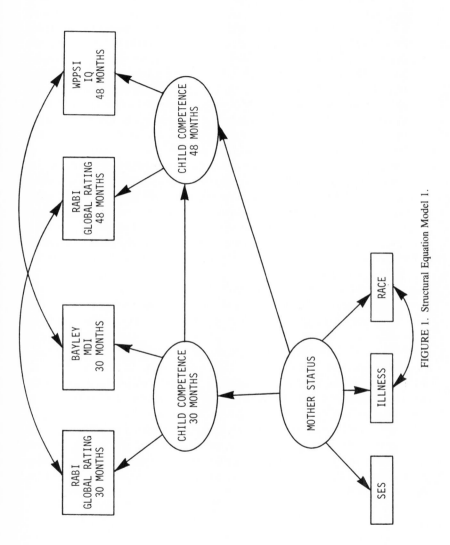

FIGURE 1. Structural Equation Model 1.

91

quite discrepant from the actual correlations. Second, the direct path from child competence at 30 months to child competence at 48 months is not significant, while the paths from mother status to each of the child competence variables are significant.

A second model was then defined, designed to eliminate the problems identified in Model 1, and tested. Model 2 is described in Figure 2. The difference between Model 1 and Model 2 is that the latter eliminates severity of illness from the model as well as the direct path from child competence at 30 months to child competence at 48 months. This second model was tested and found to be adequate, i.e., the chi-square statistic is small compared with the degrees of freedom and does not approach significance (chi-square = 5.29, df = 5, .30 < p < .50). Also, the hypothesized causal paths. among variables are significant.

Because this result is surprising , i.e., there appeared to be no direct influence of child variables in the continuity of competence, a third model was tested. Model 3 differs from Model 2 in that the direct path from child competence at 30 months to child competence at 48 months is restored (see Figure 3). This model was tested and, like Model 2, was found to be adequate; the chi-square statistic is low and does not approach significance (chi-square = 3.60, df = 4, .30 < p < .50). However, there are two factors that qualify this assessment. First, as in Model 1, the direct path between child competence at the two ages is not significant. Second, Model 3 is not significantly better than Model 2 in explaining the data. A simple chi-square test of the difference between Model 2 and Model 3 is not significant (chi-square = 1.69, df = 1, .10 < p < .20).

From the analysis of these three models the most parsimonious explanation for the relationship between child competence at 30 and 48 months is the stability of background variables, in this case social class and race. Although a model hypothesizing a direct causal effect from competence at the first point in time to the second also has an acceptable fit to the data, it lacked two important properties. First, the addition of this parameter does not significantly add to the adequacy of the model. Second, the added parameter is not itself significantly different from zero. Thus, one follows the traditional bias in favor of the simpler of two conceptual models when the choice is ambiguous.

Implications for Prevention

The analysis we have attempted in this report is based on an understanding of the developmental process which centers on both the developing child and the environmental context in which that growth is taking place. Recent

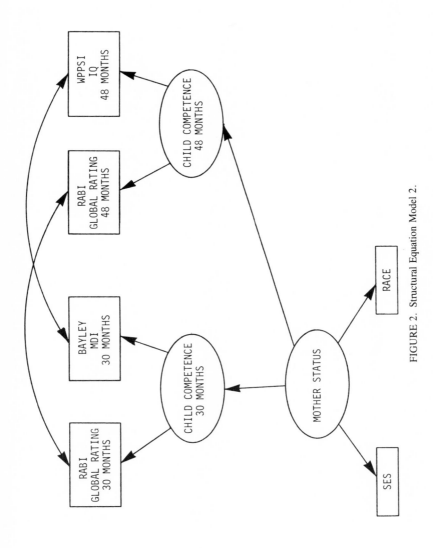

FIGURE 2. Structural Equation Model 2.

93

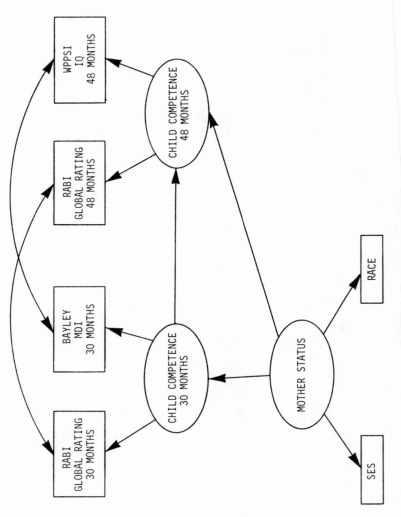

FIGURE 3. Structural Equation Model 3.

94

clinical research in areas such as schizophrenia or hyperactivity, as well as the development of intelligence, has placed great emphasis on constitutional contributors to behavior (e.g., Gottesman, 1978; Jensen, 1973). Although such hypotheses are appealing because they allow one to believe that the disease can be isolated from family and culture and treated in its own right, this medical model (Engel, 1977) does not fit the facts. No developmentalist would argue that there are not continuities in the child, where current functioning is built upon the basis of prior achievements; the cliché that one cannot run until one can walk is quite true. In more modern psychological theory, one cannot engage in complex logical thought until one has passed through stages of sensorimotor and concrete thinking (Piaget, 1950). But, the evaluation, and modification, of individual differences presents additional complexity. Because one must pass through stages of development, it does not mean that the relative performance levels in later stages will be based on the performance levels in earlier stages (Sackett, Sameroff, Cairns, & Suomi, 1981). To make an analogy, strong bricks contribute to the possibility of a strong house, but if the mortar is weak, the house cannot stand. In the context of child development, the mortar in question is the new experiences the environment provides that allow the child to move to more developed levels of functioning.

In our analysis of the relations between the child's competencies at 2-½ and 4 years of age, we were able to compare the contributions to the four-year outcomes from the earlier competencies of the child with the contributions from the social and family context; that is, to compare the contribution from the bricks with the contribution from the mortar. The variables we used were relatively well established and simple to measure. The comparison of various models indicated that the most parsimonious explanation of our data was that the variations in children's performance at four years could be better explained by the background environmental variables than by the child's previous performance.

From the perspective of intervention strategies, this is an optimistic conclusion. The course of the child's development in the preschool years is significantly related to the environmental context. The primary limitations on developmental progress do not necessarily lie in the child, but may also inhere in the caregiving system which fosters that child. The results of our analysis point out a course for future research and applications, that is, to identify the components of the system related to social status and race that impede or foster the cognitive and social competencies of the developing child.

REFERENCES

Engel, G. E. The need for a new medical model: A challenge for biomedicine. *Science*, 1977, *196*, 129–136.

Golden, M., & Birns, B. Social class and infant intelligence. In M. Lewis (Ed.), *Origins of intelligence: Infancy and early childhood*. New York: Plenum, 1976.

Gottesman, I. I. Schizophrenia and genetics; Where are we? Are you sure? In L. C. Wynne, R. L. Cromwell, & S. Mathysse (Eds.), *The nature of schizophrenia; New approaches to research and treatment*. New York: Wiley, 1978.

Hanson, D. R., Gottesman, I. I., & Meehl, P. E. Genetic theories and the validation of psychiatric diagnoses: Implications for the study of children of schizophrenics. *Journal of Abnormal Psychology*, 1977, *86*(6), 575–588.

Hollingshead, A. B. *Two factor index of social position*. Unpublished manuscript, Yale University, 1957.

Jensen, A. R. *Educability and group differences*. London: Methuen, 1973.

Joreskog, K. G. A general method for estimating linear structural equation system. In A. S. Goldberger & O. D. Duncan (Eds.), *Structural equation models in the social sciences*. New York: Seminar Press, 1973.

Joreskog, K. G. Statistical estimation of structural models in longitudinal developmental investigations. In J. R. Nesselroade & P. B. Baltes (Eds.), *Longitudinal research in the study of behavior and development*. New York: Academic, 1979.

Joreskog, K. G., & Sorbum, D. *Lisrel IV: Analysis of linear structural relationships by the method of maximum liklihood*. Chicago: National Educational Resources, 1978.

Kohn, M. *Class and conformity: A study in values*. Homewood, IL: Dorsey Press, 1969.

Kohn, M. Social class and schizophrenia: A critical review and reformulation. *Schizophrenia Bulletin*, 1973, *7*, 60–79.

Lewis, M., & Wilson, C. D. Infant development in lower class American families. *Human Development*, 1972, *15*, 112–127.

Piaget, J. *Psychology of intelligence*. London: Routledge and Kegan Paul, 1950.

Ragosa, D. Causal models in longitudinal research: Rationale, formulation, and interpretation. In J. R. Neselroade & P. B. Baltes (Eds.), *Longitudinal research in the study of behavior and development*. New York: Academic, 1979.

Sackett, G. P., Sameroff, A. J., Cairns, R. B., & Suomi, S. J. Continuity in behavioral development: Theoretical and empirical issues. In K. Immelmann, G. W. Barlow, M. Main, & L. F. Petrinovich (Eds.), *Behavioral development: An interdisciplinary approach*. Cambridge: University of Cambridge Press, 1981.

Sameroff, A. J. Development and the dialectic: The need for a systems approach. In W. A. Collins (Ed.), *Minnesota symposium on child psychology* (Vol. 15). Hillsdale, NJ: Lawrence Erlbaum Associates, 1981.

Sameroff, A. J., & Chandler, M. J. Reproductive risk and the continuum of caretaking casualty. In F. D. Horowitz, E. M. Hetherington, S. Scarr-Salapatek, & G. Siegel (Eds.), *Review of child development research* (Vol. 4). Chicago: University of Chicago, 1975.

Sameroff, A. J., & Seifer, R. The transmission of incompetence: The offspring of mentally ill women. In M. Lewis & L. A. Rosenblum (Eds.) *The uncommon child*. New York: Plenum, 1981.

Sameroff, A. J., & Zax. M. In search of schizophrenia: Young offspring of schizophrenic women. In L. C. Wynne, R. L. Cromwell, & S. Mathysse (Eds.), *The nature of schizophrenia: New approaches to research and treatment*. New York: Wiley, 1978.

Seifer, R., Sameroff, A. J., & Jones, F. Adaptive behavior in young children of emotionally disturbed women. *Journal of Applied Developmental Psychology*, 1981, *1*(4), 251–276.

Wapner, S., Kaplan, B., & Cohen, S. B. An organismic-developmental perspective for understanding transactions of men and environments. *Environment and Behavior*, 1973, *5*(3), 255–289.

DEFECTIVE INFANT FORMULA:
THE NEO-MULL-SOY/CHO-FREE INCIDENT

Carol R. Laskin
Lynn J. Pilot

ABSTRACT. Two soy-based infant formulas (Neo-Mull-Soy and Cho-Free) were recalled in 1979 when it was discovered that they lacked an essential ingredient—chloride. However, thousands of infants nationwide had already used the defective formulas. Many of these infants were found to be in serious states of hypochloremic metabolic alkalosis. No one knows what the effects will be on their long-term growth and development. Two women whose infant sons had used the defective Neo-Mull-Soy discovered that the Federal government had not established quality control procedures or nutrient standards for infant formulas. The two women pressed the Food and Drug Administration and the Congress to ensure the safety and quality of infant formula. Their efforts resulted in the enactment of the Infant Formula Act of 1980 which sets nutrient standards for all infant formula and, for the first time, requires routine testing by manufacturers to ensure that each infant formula meets these nutrient standards.

On August 2, 1979, the Syntex Corporation of Palo Alto, California, recalled its two soy-based infant formulas, Neo-Mull-Soy and Cho-Free. The problem with the formulas surfaced in the summer of 1979 in Memphis, Tennessee, when three babies were hospitalized with a suspected diagnosis of Bartter's syndrome.

Dr. Shane Roy, the attending pediatric nephrologist, had tested the babies and found them to be in a state of metabolic alkalosis, an electrolyte imbalance that causes weight loss, dehydration, vomiting, and a general "failure to thrive." However, Dr. Roy knew that it was statistically impossible to find Bartter's syndrome, a very rare kidney disorder, in three unrelated individuals within such a short period of time. Then he discovered that all three babies were using Neo-Mull-Soy.

The babies' blood tests indicated a dangerously low level of chloride. Dr. Roy then tested the formula itself and discovered that Neo-Mull-Soy contained less than 2 milliequivalents of chloride per liter, even though the Physicians' Desk Reference listed the chloride content of Neo-Mull-Soy as 9

Reprints may be obtained from Carol Laskin, 2723 Devonshire Place, N.W., Washington, D.C. 20008.

milliequivalents per liter. However, the American Academy of Pediatrics recommended that synthetic milk substitutes contain from 11 to 29   milliequivalentsiof chloride per liter. Thus, Neo-Mull-Soy had less than one-fifth the minimum needed for proper growth.

Dr. Roy immediately notified Syntex and the Center for Disease Control (CDC) in Atlanta, Georgia, of his findings. Within a few days, using its nationwide list of pediatric nephrologists, CDC found 31 cases of unexplained metabolic alkalosis in children. Twenty-six of these 31 babies were using either Neo-Mull-Soy or Cho-Free.

Samples of Neo-Mull-Soy and Cho-Free produced from January to July of 1979 were then tested by Syntex. The tests revealed that all the formula contained less than 5 milliequivalents of chloride per liter. In fact, two-thirds of the cans contained less than 2 milliequivalents per liter.

At that time, Syntex was manufacturing an estimated 10% of the soy-based infant formula sold in the United States. Syntex estimated that on any given day between 20,000 and 50,000 babies were using Neo-Mull-Soy or Cho-Free.

According to Syntex, the problem with Neo-Mull-Soy and Cho-Free began in March, 1978, when the company decided to remove salt (sodium chloride) from its formulas. The decision purportedly was based on consumer pressure to reduce the salt intake of babies because of the link between salt and high blood pressure. Syntex apparently did not consider whether other ingredients in the formula would provide sufficient quantities of chloride. Moreover, the company had stopped testing its formulas for chloride in 1977. The result was the production of formulas seriously deficient in chloride from 1978 until the recall in August, 1979.

Personal Involvement

Our children were hospitalized in a state of metabolic alkalosis with suspected Bartter's syndrome in 1979. During the time the Laskins' son was hospitalized, his formula was changed from Neo-Mull-Soy to a milk-based formula, and his symptoms of metabolic alkalosis gradually began to disappear. Because there had been no other changes in his diet or any medical intervention, it became apparent that his problems might be related to the Neo-Mull-Soy formula.

In early July, 1979, suspecting that there might indeed be something wrong with the formula, we called the Food and Drug Administration (FDA) in Washington, D.C., to ask if there had been other complaints about Neo-Mull-Soy. In the course of our conversation, we asked about the testing requirements for baby formula. We were told by several FDA officials that there were only two requirements for the manufacture of baby formula: (1) the formula must be manufactured under sanitary conditions, and (2) the label must reflect what is in the can. There were no up-to-date requirements concerning the nutrient composition of the formula, nor were there requirements for quality control procedures to ensure that the formula contained the ingredients that it was intended to contain.

Upon learning of the recall of Neo-Mull-Soy and Cho-Free on August 2, 1979, we were firmly convinced of the link between the formula and our children's problems.

At first, the FDA, Syntex, and the Center for Disease Control concentrated their efforts on removing the defective formula from the marketplace and communicating simple, basic information to pediatricians and distributors. Unfortunately, both the FDA and Syntex handled the problem as a routine matter with very little effort to ensure the effectiveness of the recall, or any real concern about the epidemiology surrounding the incident or its long-term effects.

It was of especially great concern to us that, despite the recall, the deficient formula was still readily available in many local supermarkets and pharmacies. Our concern and disappointment reached the action point when we discovered supplies of the defective formula on retail shelves 2 months after the recall had been initiated. We contacted the FDA repeatedly to report the name and location of stores that were still selling the deficient formula. We asked FDA officials how a similar incident could be avoided in the future given the lack of nutrient standards, quality control regulations, and the obvious ineffectiveness of the Neo-Mull-Soy/Cho-Free recall. We received a minimal response. The FDA admitted that they had done a poor job in handling the recall, but claimed it lacked the authority to establish nutrient standards and quality control procedures.

It was also troubling to us that despite the fact that a defective infant formula had been used by 20,000 to 50,000 infants at any one time over an 18-month period, the CDC had identified only 100 cases of metabolic alkalosis. Surely there had to be more infants who were adversely affected and who needed treatment and follow-up.

After many frustrating attempts to deal with the FDA bureaucracy, we contacted a local Washington, D.C., television consumer reporter. She did a series of television reports on us and the ineffectiveness of the Neo-Mull-Soy/Cho-Free recall and the possibility that if nothing were done, a similar incident could occur again with other baby formulas. She alerted members of the House of Representatives' Committee on FDA Oversight to watch the report on television. Within a week, on November 1, 1979, Congressional hearings were held to investigate the Neo-Mull-Soy/Cho-Free incident.

Following these Congressional hearings in the House, Congressmen Gore (Tennessee), Mottl (Ohio), and Carter (Kentucky) introduced legislation dealing with the manufacture and distribution of baby formula. Senator Metzenbaum (Ohio) introduced similar legislation in the Senate in January, 1980.

Realizing that the legislative process could take years and that there was no protection in the interim for babies using infant formula, we decided to press the FDA to change the classification of infant formula from a food to a non-prescription drug (e.g., aspirin). This approach had two major advantages over the long legislative process: (1) Since the FDA already had the authority to regulate infant formula as a non-prescription drug, there would be no need for new legislation, and (2) although the production of infant formula would have to follow the more stringent non-prescription drug guidelines, it would still be readily available to the consumer. We presented our plan to FDA Commissioner Jere Goyan on January 30, 1980.

The FDA's response was to downplay the possibility of regulating infant formula as a non-prescription drug. It appears that one of the FDA's aims was to broaden their legislative authority over the production of foods in general. Consequently, the FDA urged us to concentrate on a new law to establish a special category of food called "infant formula."

Establishment of FORMULA

Following our appearance on local television and after news coverage by the *Washington Post*, we received telephone calls and letters from other parents whose children had used Neo-Mull-Soy or Cho-Free. The parents wanted to know what symptoms our children had while using the defective formula and what problems they had now. The parents also wanted to be able to talk to someone who understood their concern, fear, and anxiety about their children.

In response to this critical need, we formed a parent-support group which became known as FORMULA.

Initially, most of the parents who contacted us were in the Washington, D.C., area. However, in March, 1980, the ABC television program, "20/20," produced a segment on the Neo-Mull-Soy/Cho-Free incident in which we appeared. We contacted ABC-affiliated stations throughout the country and informed them that parents seeking more information should be told to write our post office box. We received several hundred letters.

We forwarded a prepared package of materials to each parent who wrote. This package included four documents: a letter to parents explaining who we were; a fact sheet detailing why the formula was defective, the problems the children had while on the formula, and the problems they were having now; a four-page questionnaire asking for detailed information about the child's problems; and a list of published medical references on the Neo-Mull-Soy/Cho-Free incident for parents to take to their doctors.

Our goals for FORMULA are two-fold: (1) to ensure that the children who were on the defective formula receive the proper medical attention; and (2) to ensure that the Federal government acts to prevent incidents like this from ever happening again. We incorporated as a non-profit group and received tax-exempt status from the Internal Revenue Service.

Throughout 1980, we worked with Congressional staff members to draft a law requiring stricter control over formula manufacturing. The result of our efforts was the passage in September, 1980, of the Infant Formula Act of 1980 (Public Law 96-359), which sets nutrient standards for all infant formula and, for the first time, requires routine testing by manufacturers to ensure that each infant formula meets these nutrient standards.

We have now become the national information and resource center for parents, governmental agencies, physicians, teachers and other professionals who are involved in the Neo-Mull-Soy/Cho-Free incident. To date, we have received more than 60,000 letters asking for information about infant formula. Approximately 5,000 of these letters have asked for specific information about Neo-Mull-Soy or Cho-Free.

The Effect of this Incident on Families

Because we read over 5,000 letters specifically dealing with Neo-Mull-Soy/Cho-Free, and have already received hundreds of completed questionnaires, we are able to identify recurrent problems among these children. The major problems reported about the children consuming the defective formulas in 1978–1979 include slow gross motor development, speech delay (expressive language), kidney problems, hypotonia, convulsions, and serious dental problems.

We have also received many letters from parents of older children who were fed Neo-Mull-Soy or Cho-Free manufactured prior to 1978. It appears the formula may have been below the minimum standard for chloride for many years prior to 1978. The older children seem to have the same symptoms as the younger children. In addition, many of these older children have been diagnosed as learning disabled. Previously, many of these children had been considered for diagnoses ranging from Bartter's syndrome to cystic fibrosis and cerebral palsy.

This incident had and continues to have a devastating psychological, emotional and financial impact on all members of the children's families. We have had reports of fathers deserting their families because of the stress of a sick child, of mothers seeking psychiatric help because of the constant pressure and frustration of their child's poor health, of welfare agencies accusing parents of gross neglect or abuse because of their child's malnutrition, and of marriages ending in divorce. We have also been told of parents mortgaging their homes to pay the medical bills.

The long-term psychological effect on the children of being hospitalized, of being constantly poked and prodded is unknown. Many children saw and continue to see numerous medical specialists on a routine basis. In addition, these children are enrolled in physical, occupational, and speech therapy programs.

The anxiety surrounding this incident continues. Since no one knows what the long-term effects of chloride deprivation are on a child, the stress continues.

Positive Societal Factors

Translating what a few people believed to be a widespread problem into a national movement that would rapidly gain force and momentum was a difficult undertaking. However, there were four things that helped us: (1) our backgrounds, (2) the media, (3) the fact that it was an election year, and (4) consumer pressure.

First, each of us had some expertise in areas which could be used to accomplish our goals. Carol Laskin is a health care management consultant for a variety of clients including the Department of Health and Human Services. Lynn Pilot is an attorney with experience in Congress as an Administrative and Legislative Assistant. Alan Laskin is a management consultant with knowledge of the television, radio, and newspaper world. Larry Pilot, an FDA official for 10 years, is a practicing attorney specializing in food and drug law.

Second, living in Washington, D.C., we could meet face-to-face with FDA officials and Congressional staff. We knew where and how to obtain information from the numerous resources available to us.

Third, we discovered how effective it could be to work with the media. Because the issue of "motherhood and babies" was so appealing, the infant formula story was covered by news services, radio stations, and local, cable and national television.

As our battle intensified over the precise wording of the legislation, the *Washington Post*, the *Washington Star*, the *New York Times*, and the *Wall Street Journal* all wrote feature stories about our fight to make routine testing of baby formula mandatory. The publicity which was generated created sufficient pressure that, at the last minute, Congress agreed to include routine testing provisions in the present law.

Publicity was a particularly strong asset because it was an election year. Senators and Representatives wanted to be able to tell their constituents that they were protecting babies. Consequently, we received the support of both Democrats and Republicans.

Finally, the 1970s brought credibility to consumer participation in the political and legislative processes. We were accepted as legitimate spokespersons during FDA hearings and during meetings with Congressional staffs and were considered to represent the interests of parents across the country. Again, the media publicity helped to promote our cause and to serve notice to Congress and industry representatives that additional consumer pressure could be mobilized if necessary.

Negative Societal Factors

Our battle to regulate the infant formula industry was not without its major obstacles. Primary among these obstacles was the fact that we were individuals with our own family and career responsibilities, pitted against the government and a multi-million dollar industry.

Although the Infant Formula Council (IFC), which represents the five U.S. manufacturers of infant formula, supported the principle of infant formula safety, they opposed legislation that would specify nutrient standards, quality control procedures, and testing requirements. The IFC had enormous financial and manpower resources to apply pressure and exercise influence over members of Congress and their staffs. As one Congressional staff member remarked when routine testing requirements were removed from an early version of the bill, "consumers talk to staff, drug companies talk directly to Representatives and Senators." This inequity of access could only be offset by the counter-pressures created through media publicity.

The American Medical Association (AMA) saw no need for *any* legislation regulating infant formulas because they believed the industry could and should regulate itself. The AMA took this position even after it had been revealed that there had been numerous incidents—prior to the Neo-Mull-Soy/Cho-Free recall—in which defective infant formula had been allowed to enter the marketplace.

Another problem that plagued us was access to technical experts. For example, when the drug companies commented on FDA proposed quality control regulations, they had their sizeable legal staff research and write a detailed rebuttal of the regulations. By contrast, we had to invest the time to become knowledgeable in this field. We also sought the aid of experts who would volunteer their time to help us.

Additional problems existed when we attempted to further our second goal of obtaining needed medical attention for children affected by the defective formulas. Three separate components of the Department of Health and Human Services (HHS) were dealing with the formula incident—the FDA, CDC, and the National Institutes of Health (NIH).

Communication among these three bureaucracies was minimal. We, in effect, became the transmitters of information and data from one group to the next. In addition, initially there was no clear division of responsibility among the three branches. The result was inaction rather than duplication of effort.

Finally, the American Academy of Pediatrics (AAP), which represents the nation's pediatricians, displayed a passive attitude toward FDA infant formula activities and the progress of legislation being considered by the Congress. Our attempt to get the AAP to contact pediatricians by mail to inform them of the symptoms and problems of Neo-Mull-Soy/Cho-Free children resulted in a short notice in a newsletter downplaying the significance of the entire incident. Further, the AAP, to date, has displayed no interest whatsoever in pursuing any research or coordinating any efforts which might stimulate the collection of new and useful information about this subject. This lack of cooperation on the AAP's part has hampered our efforts to inform pediatricians of the seriousness of the children's problems.

Generalizability of the Situation

From this experience, we have learned some major lessons about prevention. It is easy to review the unfortunate details which led to the identification of this problem with infant formulas and to retroactively provide observations about what should have been done to prevent it. What is more important, however, is to ask what we have learned from this experience and whether steps can be taken to reduce the possibility that human errors could again develop into a major health hazard for children.

Anyone who reads newspapers, or watches television news recognizes that history seems to repeat itself—only in a slightly different way. Consider how secure we felt at one time about children's sleepwear treated with TRIS or with the safety of certain drugs taken during pregnancy. Secure, until new information was developed to suggest that perhaps too many invalid assumptions were made by industry, government, health care practitioners, and even consumers.

As consumers, we assumed that infant formulas were safe and effective. We assumed that the government was providing regulatory oversight. We believed that our pediatricians knew what was best and that they could diagnose and treat any obvious problem relating to malnutrition. We thought that the infant formula industry was at the forefront of technology and was applying the highest standard of quality control possible to the manufacture of infant formulas. We felt that the voluntary standards organizations were constantly striving for beneficial refinement and that their recommendations were being translated into product improvements by a conscientious industry. But, we were wrong. If no one had asked questions or conducted investigations, we would have continued to live the myth that infant formulas were safe because we had no reason to believe that they were unsafe. It was with this attitude that we learned the real lesson about prevention. Nothing should be taken for granted or assumed to be true for any reason that does not flow from good science or logic.

We need to ask questions and to return to basics in those areas where technology has moved so rapidly that there is acceptance merely because there is change. The Neo-Mull-Soy/Cho-Free incident can be used again to illustrate this observation. Nutritionists, pediatricians, and scientists concerned about infant growth and development have recognized for years that chloride, one of the simplest and most abundant of ions, is essential to the very life of an infant. Unless an infant is being breast fed or is on solid foods, the only opportunity to acquire chloride for nourishment would be through consumption of infant formula. Yet, for years, Neo-Mull-Soy was low in chloride and, for nearly a year and a half, it contained essentially no chloride. How was the Neo-Mull-Soy dependent infant to obtain chloride and what would happen if she/he did not? We know the answer now. But why wasn't this important question asked before?

If good health is to be sought through prevention, then scientists and physicians in private practice, industry, and government must inquire not only about the soundness of the status quo but also about the progress that is predicated upon exacting changes in the status quo. These people have the knowledge, expertise and best opportunity to ask the fundamental questions that are natural to the successful investigator or creative scientist. When an adversary asks a question, makes a statement, or offers a challenge, the response of the person interested in prevention should be a thorough investigation rather than merely sweeping aside the adversaries' views. From

our experience, we know that the simplistic responses offered by some practitioners, industry, and government representatives that "this was an isolated
incident and we have an outstanding record" is not acceptable.

We all must be courageous and persistent enough to ask tough questions
and press for thorough investigations, so that future problems will be
prevented. If just one determined person would have been more inquisitive
about chloride and infant formulas in 1978, there would have been no need
for this article.

Conclusion

Conditions will never be the same as they were prior to the Neo-Mull-
Soy/Cho-Free incident. Based on the 60,000 letters received, the authors
believe that the American public has lost confidence in the FDA and in the
infant formula industry to safeguard them from useless or harmful products.
Parents now are skeptical about the contents of infant formula, and they are
frustrated by the responses they receive from pediatricians uninformed on
the issues. Blind trust and confidence in infant formula is a thing of the past.

Clearly, Congress can provide the necessary overseeing to ensure that a
similar incident doesn't happen again. Ultimately the real solution to this
problem is within the control of the formula industry and health professions.
If there are legitimate questions about the scientific issues that relate to infant nutrition, then the medical and scientific communities have a responsibility to debate them, seek answers to important questions and pursue a
course of scientific inquiry that will restore and enhance public confidence
in those professionals whose responsibility it is to care for children—our nation's future.

PROSPECTIVE RESEARCH WITH VULNERABLE CHILDREN AND THE RISKY ART OF PREVENTIVE INTERVENTION

Jon E. Rolf
Susan Bevins
Joseph E. Hasazi
Janis Crowther
Jeannette Johnson

ABSTRACT. The Vermont Vulnerable Child Development Project is presented as an example of community based preventive intervention research employing multiple control groups and prospective epidemiology. Discussion emphasizes both methodological issues and the pragmatics involved in choosing to use community institutions in order to study preventive interventions for very young multi-risk children living with their mentally disturbed parents. Further, a rationale is provided for anticipating and coping with the political, sociological and personality conflicts which are probably inescapable in this type of mental health research.

This report is directed at persons who may be planning to conduct research involving preventive interventions for very young children considered to be at high risk for deviant development of psychological and physical skills in the short term and some sort of psychopathological outcome in the long term. The report is somewhat unusual because we have been encouraged to present our "savvy" about community based preventive intervention research

Jon E. Rolf is Director for Prevention Research, Division of Special Mental Health Programs, National Institute of Mental Health. Susan Bevins is affiliated with the Department of Psychology, University of Vermont; Joseph E. Hasazi is Associate Professor, Department of Psychology, University of Vermont. Janis Crowther is Assistant Professor, Department of Psychology, Kent State University. Jeannette L. Johnson is a Research Psychologist at the Biological Psychiatry Branch, National Institute of Mental Health.

Reprints may be obtained from Jon E. Rolf, Center for Studies of Schizophrenia, Clinical Research Branch, NIMH, Room 10-95, Parklawn Building, 5600 Fishers Lane, Rockville, MD 20857.

The Vermont Project was supported by an NIMH grant (MH 24152) awarded to J. E. Rolf and J. E. Hasazi.

instead of presenting data from our prevention project. Indeed, for persons unfamiliar with the many problems inherent in this type of research, such a discussion of the all too real gaps between the theory and practice of prevention may well prove to be the more useful one. Readers interested in our data base are referred to other reports cited below. However, before proceeding with the discussion of the issues, a brief description of our project should provide the real life contexts from which our perspectives were formed.

Our project, known as the Vermont Vulnerable Child Development Project, was one of several which comprised the Risk Consortium.* This Consortium has been engaged for the past decade in the study of children considered to be at high risk for schizophrenia and affective disorders as a function of the presence of these disorders in one or more of their parents. The Vermont Project was unusual for the Risk Consortium in that it included, in addition to prospective studies of children of mentally disordered parents (Rolf, Crowther, Bond, & Teri, in press), both preventive interventions for normally behaving and for highly deviant high risk preschoolers (Rolf, Fisher, & Hasazi, in press) and large scale epidemiological surveys of the developmental competencies and behavior problems among preschoolers aged two to six years (Crowther, Bond, & Rolf, 1981). In attempting to combine preventive intervention and prospective risk research, the Vermont Project staff came in contact with thousands of families and their preschool or first grade children. We met and worked with these parents and children either in mental health treatment facilities, in over 30 child care centers in our county catchment areas elementary schools, or simply through repeated contacts via epidemiological questionnaires mailed to the parents at their homes.

Because the Vermont Project had these different components, it can be asked whether or not ours was a study of primary or secondary prevention. We believe that it was both. Primary prevention, in its traditional meaning, was involved in our ecological and educational daycare vs. homecare intervention studies of "normal" preschoolers in the community. Secondary prevention, in the traditional sense, was studied when our daycare competency promoting interventions were combined with individualized therapeutic

---

*The Risk Consortium is comprised of a number of independently funded but voluntarily coordinated prospective research projects. A listing of some of the original projects can be grouped according to the initial ages of their subject cohorts: *The Prenatal and Neonatal Period*: Mc Neil and Kaij in Malmo, Sweden; Fish in Los Angeles; *Infancy*: Sameroff in Rochester, NY; Marcus in Israel; *Preschool*: Rolf in Vermont; *School Aged*: Anthony et al. in St. Louis; Erlenmeyer-Kimling et al. in New York City; Garmezy et al. in Minneapolis; Steff and Asarnow in Waterloo, Ontario; Watt et al. in Denver; Weintraub and Neale in Stony Brook; *Adolescence*: Goldstein and Rodnick, Los Angeles; Mednick and Schulsinger in Denmark.

(i.e., corrective) interventions for youngsters whose risks were already being expressed in cognitive, affective, social or physical deficits in developmental skills. In these cases of actualized risk, our interventions were directed at the child and his/her family ecology as well as the significant others in the child's surrounding environment. Because our intervention program was designed as a broad-band "total push," it mixed primary and secondary models of prevention in so much that a targeted child and his/her family were never totally deviant nor normal if one examined their many domains of constantly interacting developmental competencies. Furthermore, the Vermont Project staff came to believe strongly that "secondary prevention" can be equated to primary prevention when it is applied to rapidly developing children. Our reasoning is based on a developmental point of view wherein treatment (i.e., secondary prevention of a worsening problem) during a current developmental stage can also be considered as primary prevention for many aspects of behavior which will not emerge until the child achieves a later developmental stage as a function of a number of interactive maturational processes.

The Vermont Project evolved during its four years of existence, but at all times it was intended to be an exploration of the feasibility of a community based preventive intervention research project. Given its scope, complexity, and duration, we believe that this objective was achieved for the most part, but the difficulties encountered along the way were more than we could have imagined at the start. We would like to share our analyses of these problems and the unavoidable compromises between intended scientific rigor and the pragmatics of ethical clinical practice. Presented below is an initial discussion of several significant methodological and ethical issues followed by a presentation of some practical problems which came to absorb much of our creative energies.

Foreseen and Unforeseen Methodological Problems

The rationale for combining prospective risk research and preventive intervention paradigms has been presented elsewhere (Rolf & Harig, 1974; Rolf & Hasazi, 1977), but a restatement of one major issue is relevant here. The most obvious disadvantage to the prospective risk-preventive intervention design is that by actively attempting to reduce the poor prognosis of the high-risk children through preventive intervention, the prospective high-risk data are, of course, biased (Gallant & Greunbaum, 1972). In other words, the rigorous, careful wait-and-see approach of the prospective methodology is compromised. The obvious methodological solution is to plan to have high-risk no treatment controls. However, some risk types are too rare to provide sufficient numbers of subjects. Also, when the prime risk is defined as parental psychopathology and family disruption, such "no-treatment" controls are especially problematic. The Vermont Project was able to locate a barely sufficient number of children of psychiatrically hospitalized parents of preschoolers. We were also able to identify a sub-sample of untreated but needful high-risk controls for intervention children because all the high-risk children in our catchment county area could not be offered treatment due to either the project's and community's limited resources, or due to their disturbed parent's lack of motivation to accept the treatment offered for their children. We were prepared to deal with issues of sample bias, but there were other unanticipated problems too. The families of these non-treated high-risk controls proved to be extremely hard to keep in contact with over the years as their psychopathology found expression in high mobility and evasion of bill collectors. But more importantly, as has been reported elsewhere (Rolf, Fisher, & Hasazi, in press), the high-risk matched controls who remained in the project also had "breakdowns," and we felt ethically compelled to provide them with the experimental preventive interventions. Consequently, the controls themselves became treated target subjects. We thus discovered that one needs to budget for and to follow up a much larger control group than the target subject group in our type of preventive intervention program. It follows that maintaining such a large control group is also likely to be excessively expensive in staff time and frustration.

The second methodological problem we would like to address pertains especially to prevention research involving infants and preschoolers. The problem stems from the well known extremes of intra- and interindividual variations in the rates of developmental skill acquisition over short periods of time. Consequently, one can expect difficulties in detecting which changes are due to treatment and which are due to inevitable accelerations in individual children's growth curves. Similarly, one can also expect to lose sight of a single subject's progress when using group statistical comparisons (Bower, 1969). The Vermont Project attempted to cope with our intensive but highly variable data which we gathered from our individual intervention subjects through the application of both single-subject and group design methodology. In addition, we felt compelled to conduct extensive prospective epidemiological surveys of competency and problem behaviors among normal preschoolers in the surrounding general population in order to discover the normative base rates of change in developmental disorder and recovery so that we could compare each of our individual intervention subject's progress. Thus, we came to realize that a prospective prevention researcher must be well versed in a broad range of group, single case, survey, and treatment statistical methods if the research project is to be able to prove scientifically that its interventions produced greater positive outcomes than would have occurred from maturation processes alone. This need for multiple research skills is particularly true when subjects are recruited in different developmental stages, provided with different lengths of treatment according to their individual needs, and followed across a subsequent series of developmental stages in order to prove the longer term efficacy of preventive interventions.

The methodological problems inherent in most psychotherapy research were also recapitulated in our preventive intervention research with "high-risk" preschool children. Realistically, we really could not gain complete experimental control over all intervening factors even in our "total push" or broad band intervention program. Consequently, we could never be certain whether the longer term outcomes of the intervention children were the results of our own interventive efforts or if they were the results of some unknown extraneous factors (either biological, psychological, or environmental) which occurred between the period of early identification, intervention, and the assessment of later functioning.

Another problem was encountered in designing the Vermont Project, and it can be summarized as follows. The ultimate goals of high-risk preventive intervention research are the predictability of adult outcome from childhood variables and the testing of the effectiveness of preventive interventions. However, these were too remote and unobtainable during any reasonable expectation for funding by a grants institution (Rolf & Harig, 1974). Therefore, like any other non-prevention project, we had to have operational definitions of obtainable short term goals. Consequently, the short term goals in the Vermont Project were selected as (a) the collection of epidemiological data on the prevalence, incidence, and severity of behavior disorders in pre-school aged children, (b) the creation of a risk profiling system for the purpose of identifying pre-school aged children in need of future preventive interventions, and (c) the quantification of the effects of a preschool child's rates of acquisition of developmental skills as a function of exposure to daycare or homecare settings. At the end of the project, it is ironic to realize that it was these short term goals which not only secured our funding but also provided the most easily publishable data.

Comments on the Affinity of Ethical Issues for Prevention Research

Methodologically sound preventive intervention research efforts may always prove to be enormously expensive both in dollars and staff talent, but there are also other definite risks to the staff, the children, and to their families. Some of these risks are minor, others obviously major. But any of them can be amplified by a self-appointed vigilante, the type of person whose ambition is to "protect" children and society from the presumably dangerous "meddling of research minded psychotherapists." Some of these risks which had impact on the Vermont Project's daily research efforts are presented below.

In designing the Vermont Project, we were, of course, aware that identifying a child as being seriously enough at risk to need intervention may generate either a self-fulfilling prophecy through the expectations of others or it may negatively influence the child's developing self-concept when the child becomes aware of his/her risk status. We also realized that there exists the risk that the interventions provided to a needful child may be noxious, ineffective, or that a more appropriate treatment may not fit into our research protocol. As a consequence, the Vermont Project staff developed specific steps to detect any noxious effects and to refer to other service agencies any child whose needs couldn't be served by the project staff. In our case, the most frequent referrals were for speech therapy, treatment of sensory handicaps, and the treatment of physical illnesses and injuries which resulted from parental neglect and abuse.

We came to recognize that well-intentioned interventions may preempt a child's unique adaptations to his/her parents or to the larger social environment. As a consequence, we adopted a long pre-intervention waiting period before adding any new subject. Also, we tried to terminate interventions as soon as possible and to conduct careful follow-up assessments at regular intervals post-intervention.

Another unexpected risk occurred as a function of our selecting children at risk due to disturbed parenting. We observed that including these children in our preventive intervention project may have acted to increase the child's vulnerability. This happened when project staff responded to the child's verbal (or nonverbal) disclosures about parental pathology and abuse. Indeed, during the Vermont Project, several particularly disturbed and aggressive parents punished their children and temporarily removed them from the program when our staff attempted to discuss problems of maladaptive parenting and to offer assistance.

Another type of unanticipated risk to young children in prevention research occurs when a physical disorder or psychosocial stressor leads to the development of a serious behavior disorder in a vulnerable child. In our project, we discovered that the normal peers and especially the normally behaving high risk subjects in the prevention program very readily learned to imitate these problem behaviors. This tendency toward contagion of negative behaviors was a frequent but not intolerable experience in the Vermont Project. It did necessitate including its mention in our informed parental consent form and the budgeting of staff time for corrective measures.

Among the risks to the parents of high risk children in prevention intervention projects are two related ones that were particularly important to the Vermont Project. The first of these risks is that our observations of and attempts to include parents as preventive home based intervention agents of course caused project staff to recommend changes in selected parental behaviors and family rules. These seemingly simple and reasonable changes could, if imposed on a highly stressed family, upset its precarious balance and precipitate undesirable maladaptive solutions or parental separations. As indicated earlier, becoming intimately involved with the children and their parents makes it more likely that one will observe or elicit negative behaviors. During a three year period in the Vermont Project, we detected two families where serious child abuse was active. These discoveries led to the complex chain of ethical and legal responsibilities whereby we had to report these families to the local protective service agency while attempting to provide continuing care and support for the parents and their children.

Aside from the potential risks to the children and their parents, we discovered some risks which accrue to the staff of prevention projects. Some of the risks apply mostly to projects which, like the Vermont Project, recruit disturbed parents. Our staff were threatened with physical assaults and lawsuits by a number of parents. Since these threatening parents had had previous psychiatric hospitalizations and incarcerations for assaults, these threats were taken seriously. There are risks to the project because of staff leaving for reasons of personal safety as well as losing staff who become seriously frustrated when: (a) the therapeutic goals of parents and children conflict which results in the necessity for the staff to choose sides, (b) the improvements in the child achieved at the intervention center are repeatedly undone by a pathogenic home environment, and (c) either the child, the parents, or both fail to respond to maximum preventive efforts and begin to actualize their risks in increased developmental deviations or psychopathology. With regard to this last point, a project director must be sensitive to the work load of the intervention team.

Even a quick scanning of the various risks listed above should suffice to give ammunition to anti-research minded persons and to give a neophyte second thoughts in planning a project involving young children. But from any perspective, the ironies are inescapable. There are no guarantees that even carefully planned and implemented preventive interventions will not prove particularly noxious to those who most need preventive services (i.e., the very disturbed families with the highest risk children where the researcher discovers sufficient abuse to necessitate legal action for protective custody).

Up to this point, we have been discussing general methodological and ethical issues involved in designing and conducting preventive intervention research with high risk children. However, because most intervention research with young children is carried out in non-laboratory settings (such as well baby clinics, day care centers or elementary schools), there are some very real practical dilemmas in implementing even well designed intervention strategies. The Vermont Project's experiences with its high risk preschoolers and their families can serve as examples of some of these practical problems.

Some Practical Problems in Conducting Preventive Interventions in Natural Settings

Prevention research invariably involves contact with and scrutiny by the community. In order to recruit subjects, the public, governmental agencies and service institutions must be made aware of the project and its potentials for positive and noxious effects and of its promise for the advancement of knowledge about mental health.

There are politics to be learned about preventive intervention. People tend to distrust concepts they can't understand, and those of prevention, genetic risk, pathogenic families, and the distinction between experimental and control groups are all difficult to explain succinctly to lay persons without also arousing their fears. Further, persons in public institutions are defensive and reluctant to offer the support of their office when the research involves children. Official public support for a project will not be forthcoming until the office holders have been convinced that the risks to their own careers is minimal and they have also developed a trusting relationship with the researcher through repeated personal contacts. Consequently, research projects, like ours in Vermont, are vulnerable to rejection by the community when they combine prospective field and laboratory studies of populations at risk, the detection and preventive treatment of "mental" disorders, and focus on children and families.

Veterans of community based research projects will see the statements above as truisms, but novice preventive intervention researchers can be expected to grossly underestimate the extraordinary degree of social-political skills which the project's spokesperson must possess and the endless hours of staff time which must be invested in order to generate and maintain community support. It is foolhardy to ignore either the realities of the needs for these talents or the demands in time commitments when planning the staffing, the budget and the time frame of a preventive intervention project.

One must cope with divergent therapeutic philosophies of educators and other mental health providers. The second practical problem relates to working with the staff at a typical child care center, school, outpatient or community child guidance clinic. These facilities tend to attract to their staff a wide variety of persons with divergent training. Some of these persons have chosen their careers because they believe that they will be free to create uniquely individualized services for the children under their care. Observation and evaluation of their job performance as it provides ''intervention'' for the project's subjects, or being expected to implement the research project's particular brand of treatment in their classroom or clinic settings may not only be considered by agency staff persons as undesirable, but it may also be philosophically abhorrent to them. Even worse, it has also been our experience in the Vermont Project that the directors and staff of many service institutions frequently share the attitude that children and/or society should be protected from the evils of research. Therefore, preventive intervention researchers will find it often difficult, if not impossible, to reconcile the methodology of their intervention programs with the child-rearing philosophies and adult-child interaction styles of persons staffing community service institutions. We in Vermont were unable to have our treatment programs uniformly accepted and implemented by all the staff in the day care center which we had started and were managing! This unhappy circumstance would likely be the case for any other research project which chose to use a well established service agency in the community for the site of its ''natural environment'' intervention efforts.

To illustrate several of the points introduced above, we can cite examples which we encountered with our interventions in our own daycare center for preschoolers. One pertains to our fruitless attempts to schedule regular assessment periods for our behavioral observers to rate the changes in social and physical skills of our target and control children. The observations were to occur in the ''standard'' gross motor playroom when both the targets and controls would be present. The day-care teachers were always consulted to obtain and schedule the best day in the week for each subject pair. However, there were repeated instances when the observer would arrive to find the children away on a spontaneous field trip to enjoy a change in the weather or to find the children engrossed in uninterruptable activities in separate rooms. But the most frustrating and frequent problem encountered was the substitution of free play or Sesame Street for the carefully planned doses of intervention activities. This was particularly likely to occur when a new day-care teacher refused to become part of the established research team because she wanted to regain the spontaneity of her own remembered childhood.

Mainstreaming seriously misbehaving children in a community service center can be a mixed blessing. The issue here is whether to separate already disturbed high-risk children or family groups from their normal peers when designing preventive intervention programs. Many parents and educators fear that, because modeling is a two-way street, not only will the high-risk children and families be influenced by their competent peers, but the "normal" ones will also come to imitate disturbed behavior. Said another way, preventive programs can also lead to contagion of psychopathology. This is not a new issue. In the mid-1970s there seemed to be a consensus among most workers in early intervention that the data from the special education literature indicated that selective mainstreaming was more often a positive socializing treatment for the maladjusted and seemed to do no permanent or significant harm to "normal" children. Consequently, the Vermont Project Staff chose to use its full service day care center as the natural environment wherein we could integrate some high-risk children already manifesting disturbed behavior with their "normal" peers. We did discover some negative effects of doing so, and we also came to be charged by our university's human experimentation review committee with the responsibilities of monitoring the risks of mainstreaming, helping staff correct any negative contagion effects, and informing all parents enrolling their "normal" children in the host day care center that "exceptional" children and families were also in treatment there.

Since the termination of our preschool project, Public Law 142-94 has required much larger scale mainstreaming of seriously disturbed children in public school classrooms. Teachers and principals have been understandably ill-prepared to cope effectively with the special educational and behavior management requirements of these deviant children. Today, they need and want help from competent professionals to treat the deviant and to provide preventive intervention programs for their normal classmates. Unfortunately, the school staff may not have the time to teach their courses, implement experimental treatments and keep data. Nor may they be motivated to support research which would produce evidence that mainstreaming is either cost-effective or educationally desirable. This is because many teachers resent using class time to provide "therapeutic experiences" for disruptive children or exposing normal students to deviant models. Further, many principals have been repeatedly subjected to law suits by disgruntled parents when their particular child doesn't get better in response to the special individualized education program in the mainstream. Thus, the politics of mainstreaming will undoubtedly continue to influence future prevention research, at least in the schools. It is also having an impact in prohibiting alternate approaches in more restrictive clinical settings where there are more adequate facilities and trained staff to provide the intensive, consistent interventions required by the highest risk children and their parents. This type of staff expertise and consistency of intervention is particularly important for cases in which parent training is required to create home based interventions in order to maintain the gains achieved in the clinic or school.

Dealing with difficult and disturbed parents of children in prevention programs can become a "catch-22" experience. While there is both a strong clinical tradition and a rich clinical literature pointing to the importance of parent participation in early intervention programs, the bulk of the early intervention research literature concerns the cognitive rather than social development of the child in the context of non-disturbed familes. There is very little documentation which directly specifies what it takes to conduct preventive intervention research with a young high-risk child and his/her psychopathological parents. One would anticipate that disturbed parents can present special difficulties, particularly if their own problems are severe and require a good deal of their personal resources as well as therapeutic efforts by the intervention staff.

Initially we planned the ''total push'' preventive interventions to include parental participation because many parents of intervention children were seriously disturbed themselves. However, we were unable to attract many of these parents into formal educational or therapeutic activities. Also, we found that we had to work hard to counter the parent's initial suspicions and mistrust of us as ''agency people,'' deal with the delicate balance between support of the high-risk family and concern for the child's safety in it (particularly when neglect or abuse was involved), and otherwise attempt to impress upon many parents the seriousness of their child's problems. Our project's problems with parents manifested themselves in an endless variety of ways ranging from the parents' inability to wake up on time to get their children to the day care center, to giving children barbiturates or marijuana prior to coming to the day care center, to actively resisting our project staff's attempts to teach their children new social skills, or to subjecting their children to sexual or assaultive experiences. Consequently, our intervention staff worked with numerous high-risk children during the daytime only to be frustrated when many intervention gains were undone by parents when the children went home in the evenings.

The details of the Vermont Project's experiences with parents are presented elsewhere (Rolf, Fischer, & Hasazi, in press). For the purposes of this discussion of parental involvement, it should suffice to say that the project team must decide what constitutes the minimal level of parental cooperative participation that the research protocol demands and must make the child's inclusion as a subject contingent on it. It is best to use a written contract with an explanation to the parent why such a conditional limit is necessary and ethical for a research oriented project.

Avoiding all situations where self-fulfilling prophecies could become operative is not possible in prevention research. Indeed, we were repeatedly faced with these questions. How does a preventive intervention project identify a child at risk without having this identification lead to the child's downfall via stigmatization or the fulfillment of prophecy by other persons in the community? How does one give parents sufficient information about the concepts and consequences of risk for them to provide informed consent for their children to participate in preventive intervention? How does one measure the effectiveness that a treatment (given in one controlled context) has on the child's behavioral competencies in the larger community without contaminating that community source with negative expectations? How does one inform another institution which will soon interact with a treated high-risk child in a future developmental stage (e.g., when a preschooler moves on to a public grade school) that a prevention project has an ongoing interest in the child's development without "red flagging" the child or interfering with the child's rights for future privacy? We now believe these and similarly difficult issues are inherent in prevention research. For the past decade, they have been confronted and frequently resolved by all the projects in the Risk Consortium in their respective communities. Many of them are discussed by William Curran in his thoughtful article entitled "Ethical and Legal Consideration in High Risk Studies of Schizophrenia" (Curran, 1974). The point to be made here is that the projects in the Risk Consortium have survived in the face of these issues. With thousands of children at risk from at least a thousand families with a psychotic parent participating in these projects, and with hundreds of schools providing additional social and academic competence data for the projects, there have been only one or two project threatening incidents. Even with these exceptional cases of complaint (usually an uncle or in-law of the child who was afraid of a family skeleton being revealed), the peer review investigations found that the project staff conducted themselves ethically. Therefore, one can conclude that this type of research can be done ethically and safely, but it will never be easy.

The Vermont Project handled these issues pragmatically by fully disclosing to the parents and the human research review committee members the impoverished state of the arts of prevention research including our inability to accurately predict outcomes for high risk children and the need for more basic research to learn how to match preventive interventions to truly receptive children at risk. Also, we purposefully accepted children for intervention in our project only if they were at such high risk that they were either manifesting behavior problems or who were referred to us by others because they were giving clear indications of incipient developmental deviations. In addition, we had gained a non-interventionist's perspective from what might be considered an untreated high-risk group. As previously mentioned, these were children of parents who had been hospitalized for psychological problems whom we were evaluating as part of a separate non-intervention descriptive study. Most of these children were not evidencing behavior problems. This fact helped us to be conservative in recommending preventive interventions for them as a group. However, if any of these children started showing significant developmental problems (as was the case for about ten percent of the families), we spoke to the parents and suggested that they seek appropriate professional assistance. We did this because we had formed intensive relationships and investments in many of these high-risk families. Indeed, we often found ourselves acting as surrogate parents. As such, we shared a parent's special double-bind of risking the creation of self-fulfilling prophecies by recommending our children for therapeutic services as compared to risking the consequences of not providing therapeutic services at the earliest opportunity for these apparently needful children. For the most part, our offers of referrals were well received by the recently hospitalized parents. Many, especially those recovering from depression, were concerned that their own illnesses would adversely affect their children. A separate study was conducted to examine these issues more closely and the interested reader can find more information in Rolf, Fischer, and Hasazi (in press).

Some Conclusions about the Pros and Cons of Conducting Primary Preventive Intervention Research with Very Young High-Risk Children

After listing the difficulties of doing hybrid preventive intervention research with high-risk children in natural settings, one must finally judge the desirability of encumbering oneself with a research project which has all these pitfalls.

In summing up our experiences, we of the Vermont Project would like to suggest the following checklist to anyone planning preventive intervention research with high risk children:

(a) Seek staff with exceptional abilities to interact gently and persistently with persons having divergent educational and philosophical backgrounds. These staff persons must be able to tolerate a great many delays in program implementation and in the emergence of visibly successful treatment outcomes. Professional training is of lesser importance than the endurance traits found in long distance runners.

(b) Realize that it will be an extremely expensive and complex undertaking. Federal funding agencies, local government and human services officials, medical treatment facilities, school systems, day care operators, parents, and children must all be courted and joined together with a spirit of common purpose.

(c) Be aware of your therapeutic limitations. You may be of more help to some children by referring them to other service programs or agencies. More important is the caution that there probably are some children (i.e., those with biological and environmental handicapping factors) who are at too great a risk to profit from even the most intensive and broadly defined intervention strategies while they remain in their naturally pathogenic environments. Probably it is the moderate-risk child (where the biological and environmental risks are not multiplying the negative effects of each other) who should be the target of infant nursery or day care oriented primary intervention research programs. The highest risk child with sensory, motor and intellectual handicaps and who also has a psychotic parent may be more properly considered a candidate for the type of intensive skills training program which would require specialized foster parenting.

(d) Be prepared to deal with the issue of children's rights versus parent's rights. Despite agreements concerning confidentiality, you may be forced to choose between parent's and children's needs during times of serious parental neglect or abuse.

(d) In each case selected for intervention, choose multiple control cases, some of whom appear to be vulnerable and others invulnerable. Contrast these cases especially with regard to the sources of these developmental competencies. In what ways and to what extent do they receive competent modeling from significant others in their natural environments? Expect control group attrition and crossover to the treatment condition.

(f) Keep in mind Paul Simon's developmental musical dictum that "One man's ceiling is another man's floor," i.e., that outcomes may be measured within and across the stages of development. In this way, secondary prevention during an early stage can be considered as primary prevention for a subsequent stage.

(g) Never underestimate the complexity of the definitional problems inherent in issues of competence and psychopathology in infancy and childhood. A truly skillful researcher must sample from multiple competency-incompetency domains across the stages and ages to sort out what competencies were promoted and what disorders may have been prevented.

(h) With respect to choosing treatments to call preventive interventions, one had better make a "total push" attempt lest the treatment effects disappear like a dropped stone's ripples on a windy pond. Consider the "booster dose" model at successive developmental stages as a relevant method from the public health practice of repeated innoculations against disease. Do this because no sane educator would propose that one brief academic course can insure an always educated person nor would a psychotherapist expect that a single bout of treatment would cure clients of all future mental disorders.

(i) Finally, be aware that the data analysis requirements of such a preventive interventions project will be staggering. Longitudinal multi-variate analyses with unequal N's, irregular intervals and episodically missing data will abort most conventional computer programs before they run. Similarly, the non-identicality of the same trait measures for different developmental stages makes for shifting definitions of the critical constructs of deviance and competence. Make your data analysis budget a hefty one.

(j) All in all, the Vermont Project staff believe that the pros of combining primary intervention with high-risk child research outweigh the cons. We encourage others to test the effectiveness of early interventions strategies with high-risk children, but we obviously feel that you should be forewarned of the difficulties that lie ahead.

REFERENCES

Bower, E. *Early identification of emotionally handicapped children in school*. Springfield, Ill.: Charles C. Thomas, 1969.

Crowther, J., Bond, L., & Rolf, J. The incidence, prevalence and severity of internalizing and externalizing behavior problems among preschool children in daycare. *Journal of Abnormal Child Psychology*, 1981, *9*, 23–42.

Cowan, E. Long-term follow up of early detected vulnerable children. *Journal of Consulting and Clinical Psychology*, 1973, *41*, 438–446.

Curran, W. Ethical and legal considerations in high risk studies of schizophrenia. *Schizophrenia Bulletin*, 1974, *10*, 74–92.

Gallant, D., & Grunebaum, H. *Preschool children at risk for schizophrenia: Research issues and variables*. Paper presented at the Dorado Beach Conference on Risk Research in Schizophrenia, Dorado Beach, Puerto Rico, 1972.

Garmezy, N. Vulnerability research and the issue of primary prevention. *American Journal of Orthopsychiatry*, 1971, *41*, 101–116.

Mednick, S., & McNeil, T. Current methodology in research on the etiology of schizophrenia: Serious difficulties which suggest the use of the high-risk group method. *Psychological Bulletin*, 1968, *70*, 681–693.

Rolf, J. *The risk prospects of preventive intervention for schizophrenia.* Paper presented at the Rodnick Conference—Preventive Intervention in Schizophrenia, Los Angeles, 1980.

Rolf, J., Fischer, M., & Hasazi, J. Assessing preventive interventions for multiple-risk preschoolers: A test case. In M. Goldstein (Ed.), *The prevention of schizophrenia.* Rockville, Md.: NIMH, in press.

Rolf, J., & Harig, P. Etiological research in schizophrenia and the rationale for primary prevention. *American Journal of Orthopsychiatry,* 1974, *44,* 538–545.

Watt, N., Anthony, E. J., Wynne, L., & Rolf, J. (Eds.). *Children at risk for schizophrenia.* New York: Cambridge University Press, in press.